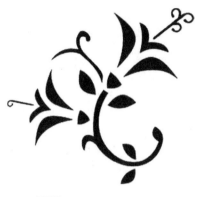

Escape

Based On a True Story

By G. V. Cora

ALL RIGHTS RESERVED

Copy/Line Editor: Robert Kidd

Final Edits &Book Design: Wicked Muse

Cover Art By: Nicolae Trifu

Dedicated to Liam Alexander Kelly.

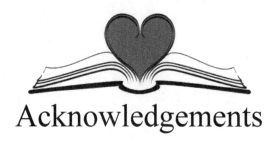

Acknowledgements

When I was halfway through writing this book, with a push of a button, I lost everything. What do you think was my reaction? To give up! Knowing this, you can imagine how grateful I am now, to those that made me start over. So, thank you to my family for insisting I finish writing.

An angel sent from Heaven, this is Leanore Elliott.
She worked hard to make my book a readable book.
Writing a book in English, my second language, wasn't an easy task.
So, that's why God sent her to my rescue. And oh boy, she did an amazing job.
Thank you Leanore Elliott, consider all existing "thank you" words and sentences in English language have been used by me.
"Îți mulțumesc" is my Romanian expression for "thank you."
Leanore, thank you.

All my gratitude to Sharon Newton for convincing me to write down this true story.

Book Description

ESCAPE... is an historical recounting of one unique family's journey of strength and love across four generations.

When the Second World War crossed Romania's borders, the changes were drastic and disorienting, transitioning from a monarchy to Communism, from a "good life" to poverty while moving through a range of emotions from love to the heavy burden of lost hope. To being asked to give up your child because of her physical handicap and ultimately, to achieving independence.

This book will take you through all the struggles, tears, and pain from the dark hell of lost love, unexpected sacrifices and a regime that nearly suffocated a once beautiful country hanging like a dark shadow above all. Come and share the journey one family took to reach the light, to survive and succeed.

Introduction

Dear Reader:

Imagine your life as a lavish, beautiful lawn, the way it was intended to be, but weeds invaded that lawn. Your entire life becomes a struggle to get rid of those "weeds" and to achieve what you deserve…a beautiful life.

By writing this book that you hold now in your hands, I extend my tribute to you.

This book will make you think deeper of your own life.

So now that you are holding my book in your hands, I would like to ask you a question: Did you say, "thank you" this morning when you woke up?

Thank you for being able to walk, talk, see, eat, hug, love—thank you for everything? Did you think about how other people are living or have lived?

After reading this book you will aim to become a better person, feel grateful for having been born in a free country, and find the strength to achieve your own independence.

Now, think about how many more reasons you have. Enjoy the journey!

Gabriela Voiculescu Cora

Prologue

LOVE...CARE

"Hold me tight, tight," Ana said to Alex, leaning her head on his chest. The moment she felt his arms around her shoulders, rivers of tears poured down her cheeks, the relief invaded each cell of her brain and covered her mind like a blanket.

Alex could feel her pain and he tried to hold her tight. Nothing in the world could make him move or take his arms away from his wife.

After a while, Ana became quieter, calmer and he let her be that way. The moment the tears came, her whole life was played like a movie only she could see...

CHAPTER ONE

Titus Salomea tried to take care of the house, the shop, and his father. His mother had passed away a few years ago and that had been hard on his father. Titus was born in a small village in the northwest part of Romania, a beautiful part of the country, a famous region providing crystal vases, glass windows, and glass art items.

From father to son, the manufacturing secrets and skills were passed down. Titus loved his work. He loved making those wonderfully delicate things. One day, he decided to move to Bucharest, the capital city, knowing he could make a good future for himself.

His crystal vases and glass work were very well received by customers. It didn't take long for the high society of that time to notice Titus's work and send him custom orders.

Shortly thereafter, his business was booming and everybody was happy.

The shop sat right in the middle of Bucharest at "Kilometer 0." If someone asked what "Kilometer 0" meant, the answer was always…from this point in the city, all measurements in Romania start. Titus's shop was located in the heart of downtown.

Those were good times back then in Bucharest, and all over Europe. This was before World War II took hold and destroyed everything. There was still a sophisticated atmosphere, very much like in France. The architecture of the buildings brought Bucharest the name of "Little Paris." It looked so much like Paris. Because people traveled all over the world, and most of their children went off to study in Paris, the French language even became popular in

Romania. It was a happy time for everybody and for the country. The King ruled with respect for the population and people responded the same way.

Titus worked hard, being ambitious to become a well-situated gentleman. He had no intention to start a family, but one day, he noticed a young girl who took his breath away.

She was petite, with dark hair and brown eyes.

Nothing extraordinary, but Titus felt like lightning had struck his heart!

He had to find out who the girl was, her name, where she lived —everything!

Titus didn't want to scare her. She looked so young.

A couple weeks later, Titus saw the beautiful girl again. She was accompanied by a man and a woman. Titus assumed they were her parents. They were coming out of the same church Titus attended. Now that he knew he could see her at his church, he made a plan to be there every Sunday and he would find a way to be introduced. After all, he couldn't just walk up and spout out his name. He went to church almost every Sunday anyway, but now it was his mission not to miss even one Sunday.

Finally, one Sunday, Titus noticed a person he knew talking to the girl's family. He couldn't be happier. The person was one of his customers and Titus couldn't wait to talk to him. As soon as he finished talking to her family, the girl and her parents left the church. Titus walked casually toward his customer, but his anticipation spilled over and he spoke in a rush, "Hi, George. I am so glad to see that you come to the same church I do. I have to ask you a big favor." Titus didn't let the man say even one word. "I noticed a few minutes ago you were talking with a gentleman. There was a lady, too, and a beautiful young girl, that I think is their daughter."

"Yes, you are right, and I see where you are going...Do you know them?" asked George.

"No, but I want to. I think I'm in love with that girl," said Titus eagerly.

"Oh, take it easy! You said you don't know the family, so how can you love the girl?" George asked.

"I don't know, but I know I love her. Please introduce me to her, and I will do whatever you want me to," Titus pleaded.

"A few crystal vases will do it," the customer said, smiling. "You know how much my wife loves your stuff. Titus, the girl is smart, beautiful and she is a good girl. Let me talk to her father and if he agrees to meet, I will let you know. Start working on my vases," he said, waving his hand and smiling as he walked away.

Next Sunday, Titus watched closely as George approached the girl's family and spoke to the father. They all turned their heads to look at Titus.

The girl's gaze met Titus's eyes for a fraction of a second and the world disappeared. In that fleeting moment—was everything. It sealed their fate.

Nora's father, Nora was her name, had to touch her arm to bring her back to reality. Even her father was impressed by Titus.

Tall, handsome, gorgeous, elegant, stunning, and most of all, he looked like a real gentleman. In his mind, he had already agreed with Titus. One single moment can change somebody's life. One of those moments, that needs no words because it cannot be described.

George waved and asked Titus to come closer.

Titus was still in shock but tried to walk straight and tall. He was introduced to everybody, and when he slowly raised Nora's hand and gently kissed it, he was lost in dreams.

Nora's father realized the moment was special and tried to have a conversation, but it ended all too soon. "Nice to meet you," he said. "See you next Sunday."

The family left the church and Titus stood there, counting the seconds until next Sunday would come.

* * * *

The week seemed to go on far too long, and when the day finally came, Titus was there first, waiting for the doors to open.

His eyes were like search lights, scanning, rotating, looking everywhere. His intense gaze screamed out his love.

Nora and her family finally arrived.

Titus's heart was beating so fast and loud, he thought people could hear it. They greeted each other and Nora's father, David, invited Titus to join them, to stay together. After the service, they exchanged a few words and said, "Goodbye and see you next Sunday."

Next Sunday came, followed by another Sunday and another Sunday. During each, Nora and Titus began getting to know each other by exchanging just a few sentences, but their eyes were talking for both of them, having long conversations full of love. There were kisses and hugs, joy and hope in just their eyes!

Love's flames were so bright even a blind person could see them. Nora's family liked Titus, the way he behaved, the way he treated their daughter, the respect he showed for them as parents. Titus was so serious and dedicated to his work and this made a solid impression on Nora's father. He already thought this young man could build a safety net for his girl, who he loved so much.

Nora's parents, David and Linda, knew what was coming and they were ready for it.

Nora was allowed to see a movie with Titus and sometimes, to take long walks. Back then, there was a unique boulevard lined with linden trees, and the aroma of those trees was so amazing that people were taking long walks just to breathe it in. There were benches along the avenue inviting couples to sit and relax. There was so much love under the linden trees. Those trees had big golden flowers and their branches were getting together to form an accolade. What beauty. Nora knew she would treasure those moments forever. Her love would always cling to that aroma.

* * * *

Titus waited to ask Nora to marry him; he wanted to be sure she felt the same way he did. One day, he broke the silence and, looking in her eyes, he said, "Are you ready to be my wife? Do you love me? I want you to be mine forever."

Nora already had so many butterflies in her stomach that she couldn't say one word.

"Do you?" Titus asked, becoming anxious.

"Yes, I'm ready, and my love for you cannot be put in words," Nora finally answered. "Titus, I love you. I loved you from the first moment I looked into your eyes."

In that moment, the earth slipped from under their feet. They were so lost in each other's eyes, they couldn't have answered the simplest question. A sweet feeling of love hugged them. Titus kissed Nora's hand and covered her face in kisses. Their very first kisses.

When they arrived at Nora's home, Titus asked to see her father. He wanted to ask for his permission and his blessings.

David greeted him with a strong handshake and a welcomed hug. "Titus, Nora is my little girl and the last one to get married. I still have her in my house and she is our joy, our happiness. She will be yours now. Protect her with your mind and your body, make her happy and give us many grandchildren. You are our son now, and we love you like our own son. Be blessed and we wish you a 'brick house,' meaning that your marriage will last forever."

Titus hugged his new parents, feeling so happy. He knew he would call them "parents" from now on. He knew he was going to take good care of them, with love and devotion.

* * * *

Nora was waiting in another room alone because her mother joined her father when Titus asked for blessings. She couldn't wait for the door to open and see everybody's happy faces. Nora loved her parents so much. They gave her love and care and she was already feeling sorry, knowing she'd have to leave them and move in with Titus.

When she saw Titus's face as he entered the room, her body was shaking, full of happiness. She kissed Titus with a kiss that seemed to last forever.

These were good times, a prosperous economy, and it wouldn't be a problem to have a sumptuous wedding, but Nora wanted to have a modest one.

It was an unforgettable wedding because of their love, which gave such an aura to everything they touched. Family and friends blessed the newlyweds with gifts and good wishes. They didn't forget to invite the man who helped Titus become the happiest man on Earth: George, the client that introduced Titus to Nora's family.

"Congratulations, I love you so much!" Maria kissed her sister and couldn't stop saying how good-looking Titus was.

"What about your husband, John? Isn't he handsome?"

"Yes, he is, and I cannot imagine my life without him, but what I am trying to say is that Titus is the best man for you."

"Silly you. Isn't he handsome?" Nora asked. "Don't think I married him for his looks. Even if I have to admit, it was the first factor when I looked in his eyes, but the way he makes me feel about everything made me think and decide he was the one, the only one."

"You made the right decision," Maria replied. "There are things in life that you just know are right. What a blessing. I was wondering if you would ever get married."

"What do you mean? Am I that old, or ugly?"

"Oh no, but this society is wrong—when it considers a woman old who is only twenty years old! And you, being twenty-two, were considered old."

"Do you think that's why our parents invited Titus to join us in church? Now I see it."

"Parents are always right. No, this wasn't the reason. Our parents saw it right away. They noticed Titus's qualities, and being so handsome helped too."

"Your husband is handsome too."

"I agree, but in a different way. Yours is just a 'movie star'!"

"Maybe he is a movie star, but a movie star that loves me with all his heart."

"Everybody can see this." Maria hugged her sister with love. "Ok, now I have to go and help one of our neighbors to deliver her baby. I will see you later, and if I have the time, I will help you decorate your new home." With that, she left.

Maria had a passion for babies and this guided her decision to become a midwife. For that, she was a really good one. Because she was only two years older than Nora, she worried people would not trust her to deliver their babies, being that young.

But Maria had a way of convincing those ladies she would do an excellent job.

Her reputation was spotless. Back then, not too many women worked. Maria didn't have to work either but she wanted to.

The satisfaction from her work was worth more than the money. Sometimes she wasn't paid at all. Not everybody she helped had her family status. There were poor women, with no money, but Maria helped them anyway. She helped everybody, with or without money. If somebody would knock at her door in the middle of the night and ask for help, Maria would go and do the best she could. Her reputation became famous in town, and women asked her to put their names on her waiting list, as soon as they knew they were going to have a baby.

When Maria came back, she looked tired.

Nora saw this and said, "Come inside and sit down. I will make you a tea and rub your shoulders." Nora rubbed Maria's shoulders and noticed her head was tilting already. She fell asleep right there on the chair. Nora covered her sister with a warm blanket and stayed close to her, thanking God for having such a sister.

* * * *

David and Linda, Nora's parents owned a large yard with two rows of houses. The main house had a large basement underneath, as long and wide as the yard was.

Maria lived on one side with her husband and their son, Peter.

Next to Maria's home was another house that was empty. Their father kept it that way, saying that they had to keep that house empty for bad days. Just in case they had to rent it, if times got harder and they needed that money to survive.

Everybody knew their father planned things for a reason. He knew that getting older, he and his wife would need help and having the children closer would benefit everybody. The grandparents could help with the grandkids and the daughters could help their parents. Being a family, a large and loving family, meant a lot to

Nora and Maria's parents.

After the wedding, Nora found out that she and Titus would live in the house that had always been empty. She couldn't believe her father's plans and how thoughtful he was.

Of course, Titus could afford to have a nice home for his bride, but it was nice to be together, to have a family. How could somebody be that lucky? Titus thought. To be married to the woman he loved and to have such a family. *God, thank you, and I promise to treasure all of the gifts you gave me. I promise.*

Nora and Maria decorated the new home and it looked amazing. The young couple moved in and each day brought more joy and happiness.

* * * *

Nora was busy visualizing her future. She could see herself asking Maria to help her deliver her babies; many babies. That day would come, hopefully soon!

Maria's son, Peter, was absolutely handsome. His eyes were so expressive; they seemed to know everything. Compared to his young body, those eyes were the best tool he could have. He could communicate with his eyes better than talking. Nora was very attached to him. They spent time together, playing and going places.

God, do you think I am too happy? Nora wondered. Do you think I will ever have a son like Peter, my nephew? I want to have a boy first, and a girl after. Ok, I will stop now. I think I'm asking way too much. Not only that I ask you for children, but I even dare to ask for a boy first, then a girl. Nora, be humble and don't forget God knows better what you need, when you need, how much you need, etc. Health is the most important thing, boy or girl. Pray for health, Nora, pray for health and peace. Be patient and wait for that miraculous time to come in your life.

She looked around the room and found lots of things to do, to keep her mind busy. *I think I should learn something new that will keep me busy and bring extra money home. Titus will think I am crazy. I don't have to bring an extra income; he can provide all the necessary things. Everybody will be against my decision, if I decide to go to school and study for something new. I know how blessed I am to be able to stay home, to have a good husband that loves me and who spoils me with flowers, jewelry; and I can hear voices saying how spoiled I am. It is not about this; it is that I have this desire to learn, to help Titus with his shop. When I wake up, the first thing that comes to my mind is school! But I think I have to pay more attention to all the events that have happened around the world.*

World War II started to spread its gray, ugly wings all over Europe. There were noticeable changes everywhere you looked. Nora hoped these changes wouldn't touch her and her family. That they wouldn't touch her city.

She tried not to think about this too much, so she focused on her goal, going to school. None of the women in her large family went to work, but when Maria became a midwife, Nora knew she would be the next to go to school. She loved figures!

Mathematics was an easy subject for her to understand and to work with. Her grades reflected her passion. One day, when she could hold her desire in no longer, she told Titus she had something to talk to him about. She started sharing her plans to go to school and learn accounting with Titus. He smiled first, but his eyes became bigger than she ever saw them. He thought this was a joke, but Nora had a serious face and was not kidding. As she waited for her husband's answer, the world disappeared, time stopped.

Titus put his arm around his wife's shoulders, looked in her eyes, and asked, "Why? Do you think this will make you happier? Aren't you happy with our life, with me? Why? Why? I have more whys, but first answer me and tell me what made you think this way? I feel so guilty now."

"Oh no, please, please, I love you so much. Don't even think it is you! No, I'm happy with you and my life. I am happy being your wife. But look around us, the war is coming closer and closer, and it seems like it has no end. We have to be prepared and face it. I know I can do it and I can help you with the shop."

"What about babies? They will come and keep you busier than you can handle."

"I know and I pray for this every day that God will take care of us. When the babies do come, our parents, like we like to say, will help a lot to raise them. They cannot wait to see those babies and me too. What a blessing to have parents like ours, still strong and healthy and so close to us; we are so blessed. I can learn something new till that time comes. Am I spoiled?"

"Yes, you are, but my love for you won't let me see you unhappy."

"Don't say this, I am happy, but I feel I have a calling and I promise, nothing will change between us."

* * * *

Titus knew by now how determined his wife was when she put something in her mind. He wanted her happy, but he hated the thought of his wife being out in the "jungle" without his protection. It was a different kind of world; one Nora has never had to deal with. He was holding her body close to his and millions of thoughts were galloping in his mind.

Suddenly, he realized he was jealous! The thought of other men around her, such as teachers, students—all different influences. Titus tried to send those things out of his mind, feeling ashamed for just thinking of it.

I trust my wife; she would never do something wrong. Yes, I want her home. Yes, I want her safe, but if finding something else to learn and doing that makes her happier, how can I dare to stop her dream? I'm selfish! Nora feels and she knows times are different; they are changing, slower, but still changing. We have a good life; we love each other so much, and if she wants to do more, it should make me proud of her. Of course, our friends and neighbors will think I cannot afford to provide enough, but they did the same when my sister-in-law went to school to become a midwife, and look now, everybody needs her and you can see how happy she is. Maybe Nora saw this before I did. Oh, women always have a special, strange something that they call intuition! I never understood exactly what it was all about. But I can see the end results. Titus turned Nora's body towards him with so much love and care that she could fall asleep standing right there in his arms. "Nora, let's sit down and talk."

Nora's eyes revealed her happiness, and she realized her victory. She knew these kinds of things don't make men too happy.

"So, you want to help me with the shop? Becoming an accountant, you will be in charge of all our money. You are anyway; why go to school for this?"

"I will be a good accountant, because I love it."

"I want to see the happiness in your eyes; I want to see your eyes looking at me with love, like you did in church. This is something I won't ever forget. So, yes, go to school. I know you don't need my permission; you're too independent, and I appreciate the fact that you asked me first. I love you so much."

Nora hugged her husband and she smiled all the way to the end of the evening. And the evening came with love and kisses.

* * * *

The next day started with so many plans and questions for Nora. She had to find a school that would accept women. She had to tell her parents about her intentions. Nora knew what their reactions would be.

Her mother always took care of the house and her children. She didn't know anything else. Her mom was an angel, loving and protecting her family like an eagle. She would think Nora wasn't happy and possibly blame Titus. How could Nora convince her mother that this wasn't about Titus, but her wanting to go to school?

On the other hand, Nora's father was different from her mom. He always let his wife to do whatever she thought was necessary to be done for the children and for the house. When the children came into their lives, he acted like a grandfather, spoiling his children as if they were grandchildren. He was so different than other men they knew. The role of the head of the house, he transferred on his wife. Providing and loving was his motto and he accomplished his mission really well. Nothing was missing in his children's lives. The way he loved his family became proverbial. The kids knew where to go to ask for things.

Her mother was tough but loving. Her rules were clear and she raised her children in harmony. The way she expressed her love was different, spoiling the kids with food she knew they loved or making sweaters and clothes to keep them warm and looking good.

The kids knew they should always be on time for dinner because their mother never called twice. They learned the rules at a very young age and they obeyed them.

One more day passed and Nora found herself postponing sharing the news with her parents.

* * * *

Titus came home earlier than normal that day. He closed the shop to go home and take Nora for a nice time together, to spend more time with his wife. The carriage was pulled by two magnificent horses and a white blanket covered the seats. He held a huge bouquet of flowers, got out of the carriage, and ran towards Nora, saying, "I wanted to spend more time with you before you start school."

In the very next second, he realized the storm he just created. Nora's eyes were as big as the flowers' bulbs. His mother-in-law's face turned pale, but she didn't say one word. Nora's father was quiet and he tried to look like he didn't hear anything.

Titus grabbed his wife and got in the carriage. When they were far enough from the house, he looked at Nora and asked, "You didn't tell them yet? Am I right?"

Nora couldn't talk. She blamed herself for not telling her parents about her plans. She didn't want to hurt them. "I'm so sorry. I should have told you that I didn't talk to my parents about the school yet. Why do I feel this way when I know how good my parents are? I'm stupid, but I want to protect them from being shocked."

"Does Maria know?"

"Yes, she does and she's even happier than I am. I had no chance to thank you for these beautiful flowers; you know how much I love them, and you!" Nora kissed her husband and all the worries went away. Their love made the road shine like it was a full moon. What a beautiful night, what a ride they had.

When they arrived home, the house was dark but they knew Linda was waiting for them with warm food, as she liked to do. Even if she knew they weren't hungry, she still wanted to give them good food.

Titus knew exactly what to do when he saw Nora's mother waiting for them. He said good night, thanked her for the food, and went in his house to wait for his wife but not before whispering in her ear, "I love you." He felt sorry for Nora, for what she had to go through, but at the same time, he knew how good her parents were.

* * * *

Once the door was closed, Nora started telling her mom about her future plans.

After a while, Nora asked her mother, "So, what do you think about my plans?" She felt sure she would hear things like: *You will bring shame to our family; people will think we have no means to live; nobody's wife goes to work but you and your sister. What kind of children have I raised, etc., etc.* So, Nora was taken by surprise by her mother's reaction.

"I'm so proud of you. I always wanted to do the same thing, but I was buried by rules, traditions, and life. Do what your heart and your mind are telling you to do. I will help as much as I can and when the time comes, when the children get here, you know what I mean, my life will belong to them." They hugged each other like never before, saying good night.

Nora was so touched by her mother's soft side. It was the first time she could read her mother's heart; the first time she could see her soul.

Titus had been waiting for his wife, expecting to see her face covered in tears. When Nora opened the door, Titus looked shocked to see the happiness across her face. She never looked so beautiful, so radiant.

Nora took her husband's hands and said, "I have the best parents in the world, best husband, best family, and best of everything."

"How was it? What did she say?"

"To go to school and be happy."

"We do have the best; let's thank God for all we have and be grateful."

Getting ready to go to bed, their minds were still floating around, but they had to get ready for tomorrow. Love filled the room and the smell of flowers conquered their dreams.

* * * *

A few months passed. The war was more and more visible. You could see the damages caused by the bomb raids. Nora was making good progress with her accounting courses. Nobody could understand why she chose accounting! It was such a "man's field." Why not something feminine like fashion, jewelry, or clothing? But this is what she liked and this is what she'd chosen. It seemed she was good at it.

One day, she asked her husband, "What do you think if I help you at the shop? I can do your books and help you do things that need to be done."

"Ok, feel free to come and do everything you want."

"No, I will do everything you tell me to do."

"Maybe for few days you will, but after that, you will discover what you want and that's ok with me. I know the shop will look much better and the customers will be happier. It will have the woman's touch that I could never offer."

"Ok, I will get ready and will make your shop a real jewel."

"You see, you've already started. I am happy and 'our shop' will become the talk of the town."

Nora put her taste and knowledge to work. The shop looked beautiful before Nora came to work there. The shop was a fashionable place with crystals and art items made by Titus and others imported from all over the world. But Nora made things sparkle like diamonds. Fresh flowers and a discreet fragrance were greeting customers whenever they entered the shop.

Titus thought he wouldn't be comfortable working together with his wife, sharing the same space, but there were hours when he couldn't see or hear Nora. My God, she was so quiet and so distinctive. Everybody that entered the shop had the most beautiful compliments for his wife.

CHAPTER TWO

"Titus, give me your hands!" Nora grabbed Titus's hands, holding them in front of her heart, and said, "I'm pregnant; I'm pregnant! I am so happy!"

The world, the house, everything was turning around for Titus. The word 'happiness' wasn't enough to explain his feelings. He thought he was a strong, athletic man, but these three words made him feel so weak. "Are you sure? Let's tell everybody, now, let's go!"

Nora followed him and they started spreading the good news. Blessings were falling from the sky for the baby, but bombs were hitting the ground too! Not close to the city, but close enough to take the joy away from people. God was looking down at his children with love and watching for their safety. More and more the landscape started changing.

Nora kept going to the shop, and when her time came closer, she started arranging things so the baby would have whatever was needed. She wanted her baby to come into this world in harmony and love. The only thing missing was the peace, the freedom of the country, what the following days would hopefully bring.

The moment arrived and a healthy, handsome boy was born. Maria almost forgot about her duties looking at her precious nephew. She couldn't believe his hair, the color and how much he had, and his big eyes.

Ok, Maria, get real; do your job, she thought. She shook her head to focus on what she needed to make Nora feel better.

After just a few minutes, the baby was in Nora's arms. The love a mother has for her baby cannot be described. Nora thought that something miraculous was running through her veins, all over her body. When she held the tiny body close to hers, on her chest, she could feel a special bond wrapping both of them together, making them one, one human being.

If anyone would have asked Nora what her name was, in that moment, she wouldn't have known it. But she knew exactly what her son's name was...Bob. "Maria, thanks for helping me so much. Now I know what women go through. Now I know how they feel, but you forget about all those things when you hold your baby in your arms. God, thank you. What a feeling."

"Yes, I thought my son, Peter was the most beautiful baby boy, but your son tops everybody. Bob is absolutely beautiful. Congratulations and all the best wishes."

Nora's mother was cleaning up and putting things where they belonged so her grandson would be greeted properly. She came inside to see how Nora and the baby were doing and to help Maria. She stopped and asked Nora how she was feeling and to let her hold the newborn.

With a large smile, Nora said, "Mom, this is your grandson, Bob, who will bring you joy. He will be a big helper around the house and my father will teach Bob everything he needs to know."

"What a day, how blessed I am to have two grandchildren, healthy and so handsome. Now I'll let you get some rest. The real life begins now. What you are going to feel, it will be out of this world; now you are a mother. I love you, my baby girl." Linda loved to call Nora her 'baby girl.' She left the room with happy tears in her eyes and ran to hug her husband.

He already knew all the details, even though he had spent most of the delivery hiding in the shed, located in the backyard, fixing things that didn't need to be fixed, and talking to God. David's prayers were only thank-you words, being thankful for all the things that had happened to him and his family. He tried to look calm when his wife found him in the shed, but his body had a tremor. Looking at her, he could see what joy and happiness could do. "Linda is still beautiful," he said to himself, "look at those eyes! After all these years, she is still beautiful, and what a woman she is."

Day by day, Bob grew up with love and care. He started to learn things and it was such a pleasure to watch him. He was discovering the world. Everybody enjoyed playing with him. He loved to kick the balls and he was quite good at it. At the same time, Bob learned how to count and he loved to play with figures. Nora knew Bob's passion for figures came from her; it was her contribution. He was arranging game pieces like an older child. He was an intelligent kid. But his favorite thing by far, was his mom reading to him, day or night.

Dr. Bitterfield, the family doctor, gave Bob's family the best health report. This doctor was their doctor for all pains, all medical issues. He was like a second father for the family.

Nora and Titus were happy, taking care of their shop and watching their wonderful son growing.

Nora prayed hard to have at least one more child, but times were getting harder and harder. People were missing the good stuff, the good food; there were fewer shops opened, fewer jobs. Even if she knew it wasn't the right time to bring a child into this world, the way it was, she still wanted to have a sister for her son.

The day came when Nora discovered she was going to have another baby. She couldn't be happier. She talked to Bob, telling him that he was going to have a baby sister! Poor child looked at her without understanding about what she was saying.

When Titus came home, Nora kissed him, telling him the news. Titus took Bob in his arms, put his arm around Nora, and started dancing and singing. Bob thought this was a new game and he liked it.

Nora's body started changing, getting bigger, but nicely shaped. Titus thought she looked so beautiful that she could be a "poster woman" for pregnancy. She kept going to work, but it was getting harder to go as often as she wanted. When there was lots of paperwork, she could often do it from home, when Bob was napping.

* * * *

Escape

The newspapers were full of articles about World War II, making people worry about their future. The peace, the sweetest thing on Earth, was shaking. The leaders of the big countries were fighting for supremacy, for power. Every leader wanted to rule over the small countries, to have them pay for his wealth and the wealth of his country, also.

The word "Communism" began to be heard more often, making people wonder how this would affect their situation, their lives. Nobody had to deal with this new form of regime before. The newspaper had headlines like: *"No more king, no more rich people, we want syndicates, unions."* It sounded like a strange foreign language.

People around Nora were changing too. The ones that always had less became more arrogant and their body language revealed even more. The fear of uncertainty, the fear of the future was on everybody's mind. People were getting poorer. More beggars were in the streets, more people were going to churches for help with food and clothes. The buildings started lacking the care that had made them look so "Parisian." Houses needed painting; fences needed to be fixed; the streets were full of holes. Less goods on the shelves, less imported food, less of everything. Men were gathering after work and had secret meetings, more preoccupied with the situation their country was in.

Nora's husband tried to be the same as before, but it was getting harder to find extra money for flowers and all the other things he'd been doing for his wife and for his son. He used to come home in a carriage, now he used the tram or the bus. He used to change his suits all the time, now he didn't pay the same kind of attention to his look, and Nora noticed all these things.

Quiet and proud, she didn't ask him why this happened, knowing the answer.

Maria had noticed those changes, too. Being a midwife, she was entering many homes to help women to deliver their babies. It seemed like there was no happiness anymore, anywhere.

Maria and her sister looked at each other and they had a conversation without exchanging any words, simply because their eyes met. Loving each other so much, they were able to silently understand the other's feelings.

Maria broke the silence and asked, "Nora, are you ok? How is your baby doing?"

"I am ok and the baby seems to be happy in my belly. What about you? How is work? Are you tired? I didn't see you yesterday and it feels like a lost day when I don't see you!"

Maria took Nora's hands and invited her to sit down. "Let's have a cup of tea and chat a little."

"Is something wrong? You never have time to sit down, but I am glad you do now." Nora couldn't stop thinking about how hard her sister worked and how many things she was able to accomplish in such a short period of time. Her home was always clean, and her son Peter was put together all the time. His shirts and shoes were just impeccable. The way Maria cooked was almost professional. She never had culinary education, but watching her mother, she learned a lot. Nora thought God poured all the talents over her sister, and she was never envious. Nora loved Maria with all her heart.

Their neighbors were amazed that these two sisters never argued that they never had a reason to.

Peter was almost ten years old with excellent academic achievements. He acted more mature than his age, so all his friends were treating him like a boss, the leader.

When the cousins played together, Peter protected Bob like an eagle. He once stopped playing just to ask Bob if he was ok. They enjoyed playing soccer together and the whole community would get involved. Soccer was the most popular sport for everybody, young and old.

John, Maria's husband, was extremely reliable, a really good husband, and an excellent father. They were doing well financially, and he was spoiling his wife the same way Titus had Nora. She had been asking John for help when her husband wasn't home. So, when Maria asked her to sit down and talk, Nora's heart started beating faster, afraid something bad happened.

"Let me make the tea and you sit down and relax," Nora offered.

"No, let me make the tea and you sit down. You are pregnant, not me!"

"Maybe you will be pregnant too; soon, I hope."

"I wish that day would come soon, but when I see what happens around us, I am not sure I want it now."

"What are you talking about?" Nora knew the answer, but she refused to admit it. She knew the war worried Maria.

"The war is not over yet," Maria said. "We have to start moving all the provisions that we have into the basement. Better safe than sorry. We have to take care of our old parents and be sure our kids have what they need if they bomb our city. Nora, let's pray that our husbands don't have to go to war. We need them here, especially you!"

"Sister, if you ever feel like you want me to do something for us, just say it. And it doesn't matter, day or night, I will do it. You are right, let's pray that our husbands will not go to war and ask God to protect our families, our neighbors, and our country. Let's pray for the soldiers that fight for us. I am ashamed to admit that I'm happy that our husbands don't go to war; thank God, they are older than the required age. So, we are going to have two men, no, three men, if we count Peter! I wouldn't count our father—he is too old to fight—but he is a strong, brave man." Nora thought a moment, and then continued, "Maria, I have a feeling this is not the right moment to bring a child into this world, in such conditions; it is a dangerous place to have a baby and to raise that baby right. But I'm determined to do the best I can with what I have. I am thinking about what to do, so my baby girl will have the necessary nutrients to grow healthy, because this seems to be a problem now. Am I rambling? I never talk so much, maybe I'm nervous."

"Oh no, it is normal to talk like this. There are so many things to consider. Wait a minute, did you just say my 'baby girl' or it is my imagination? So strange, I keep saying this too!"

"Yes, I am going to have a girl, and her name will be Ana."

Maria looked at her sister and tears filled her beautiful eyes. "I love Ana already. She will be a fighter, perfect for the times she will be born into. But let's get organized. We have to move all our provisions in the basement. Do not lift anything heavy, promise me!

So, go to your place and gather what you think you will need, just in case."

"How are our parents doing? I didn't talk to them about what we talked about. I tried to protect them. I know they went through a lot together, but being old is hard and I want them happy."

* * * *

Titus came home from the shop and saw Nora packing clothes and food. He was wondering what happened. She hugged him and asked him to help with the packing, so they could take stuff to the basement. Thank God for that basement. Titus brought his father to live with them, to be closer, so they could help him. He went to his father's room and asked him to pack few things and to go to the basement with the whole family.

Suddenly, a horrible noise came from the outside. Titus jumped and ran directly into the street. A bomb hit the city—their wonderful city! The war was getting closer to them. Maria and her family were almost ready, and they started to put their stuff on the shelves. It was the first time they realized how lucky they were to have such a big, deep place to hide. Looking around, everything seemed so strange and so cold. This was the place where they were keeping food, flour, wine, and meats to help the families go through the winters. Nora's parents filled the shelves with almost everything they needed to survive. Everybody was thinking the same thing: *What good parents we have! Look at what they did, when and how?*

Nora stared at her mom and asked, "Did you know this would happen?"

"Yes. We have a proverb that says: 'if you don't have old people around you, buy them!'" she joked, trying to make the atmosphere lighter. "We will be ok here, and we can even help other people; there is room enough."

Day after day, things were getting worse. Nora's family was safe, as safe as you can be during a war. The bombs were changing the landscape of the city, destroying lives and dreams. Most of the buildings were down and a gray, thick cloud was covering the sky.

The kids were not allowed to go outside to play, and they were asking questions about why they couldn't play outside with their friends, why they had to stay in the basement. It was hard to explain the situation and to make them understand what "war" meant.

Nora's pregnancy was doing well, but she was missing those fresh ingredients for the baby and for herself. She was concerned that her breast milk would not be sufficient for her baby's development. Nora found herself thinking more and more deeply about this, hoping and praying that her baby girl would be as healthy as Bob was when he was born. *Why am I so selfish? How many women in my situation have nothing or a lot less than I have? What should they do, kill themselves?* The brute force of that thought struck her, and Nora knew it was wrong.

No, it is what it is and I have to deal with it. I have a very loving family and good friends; why am I so worried? I'll remember what we have been told in church, that to worry is a sin! It means you do not trust God to provide all the things you need. He knows better what you need. Nora shook her head to finally get rid of the horrible thoughts running through her mind. "Look around you and be grateful. Look how much love and care surrounds you!" She looked up and thanked God for all the blessings she had. She changed her attitude, making everybody feel better.

Maria came in the basement and anyone could sense something was going on, besides the ugly war.

"Is somebody following you? Are you ok? Why are you in such a rush?" Their mother, Linda asked.

"No, nobody is following me, but they started chasing the Jewish people in our neighborhood and we know how many they are."

"Who's 'they'?"

"The Nazis! They go inside those people's homes and take them as war prisoners. They have no place to hide. No place to go. Those families are devastated. I could see the fear in their eyes. How scared they must be. We have to do something. Who wants to go with me outside and talk to those poor people? We have to let them know they can come here and stay with us."

Nora was already up, ready to go, but her mom said, "You stay here and I go with Maria! You are pregnant and crazy. How can you imagine I would let you do this? Maria, let's wait for one of our men to come home, then we can go outside and talk to people."

"Mom, I know better how to get to my friend's homes. I delivered so many babies there. You stay here with Nora, Peter, Bob, Dad, and Simon. And I'll go." Maria didn't give anybody a chance to say one word. She was already climbing the stairs of the basement. She went outside to an absolutely horrible world. She knocked on the doors where she knew her Jewish friends lived, scared and shaking. They were scared of bombs; scared, wondering if they would still be alive the next day, or even the next second. All of them were in fear for their children's lives.

Maria was hiding, trying not to be seen by the Nazis, and thanking God for knowing the back doors of her friend's homes so well. She was able to talk with many of them. Everybody was afraid to open the door, but they recognized Maria's voice.

"Grab a few things, your medications, and use the back door when you come to my house. My whole family is there. Hurry up and come. I have to go back soon, so my family will not worry about me." She finished going to all the homes that she knew had people living there who might need help. She went back home, and headed for the basement, thanking God again for taking care of her. What a relief!

Her family was grateful to see her back.

The basement became full. The conversations were minimal and in low voices. Titus and John were going outside to bring food and whatever they could find for so many people. Thank God, the well wasn't too far away in the yard and they had a stall outside.

* * * *

A few days passed with little difference. Until their dog, that had been hidden in the shed for protection, started barking in a way that everybody recognized and knew something was going on. There was no way to look outside and see what was happening, and all of them realized the danger. The kids were sleeping, having been laid down for an afternoon nap. Something had to be done, otherwise, whoever was out there would do something. The basement's population looked at each other, frightened. Not a word was spoken. The dog kept barking. Prayers were pouring out of them all; everybody talked to God! The basement was full of Jews and Christians praying together. In stark contrast to that security, this was one of those times when the men weren't home. Titus and John were going from one place to another to find the best of anything they could find, especially for Nora.

Maria stood up, took a deep breath, looked straight into her son's eyes, and said, "Peter, I have to leave, but I will be back soon. You listen to what your grandparents tell you to do, and take care of Bob. Mommy loves you," she said, hugging her son. She started climbing the stairs, stopping halfway up to look back. Her eyes were hugging each of the people who were putting all their hopes in her right now. She could see how scared they were. Nora was holding her son's hand and, with the other hand, she was holding her belly, protecting her unborn baby.

Maria opened the basement door, stepping outside. She could see a bunch of men wearing the Nazi uniforms. These people were already in the middle of the yard, looking to get inside her family's homes. Maria recognized some of the men, and she couldn't believe they had become Nazis! Some of them had been her neighbors! They became Nazi; they enrolled with the German troops in order to protect their families and for the benefits that were coming from being a Nazi. These people forgot their country, their duties. She couldn't believe her eyes, couldn't believe what she just saw. Her attitude suddenly made her stand taller. Her voice sounded firm, yet calm. She had no idea how she would talk to these people, but she did it. "Is there something I can help you with?" Maria asked.

"Yes. We know you have Jewish people in your house."

"Why would I have Jewish people in my house? What's happened? Why?"

"We ask the questions, not you. We have an order to check your entire house and the other homes located at this address. If we find out that you have been helping Jewish people to hide here, you will be arrested, too."

"I have no idea what you are talking about, but by the way…" Maria started walking towards some of those men standing in front of her with their firearms ready to attack. She got closer to them and looked deep in one of those soldier's eyes and said, "How can you dare to come here and check my house. How can you dare to do this? Do you remember who brought your son into this world when your wife was almost dying? Who saved her life? Who saved your son?"

Maria moved to another soldier and stood firm in front of him, confronting him. "Is your memory that short? It hasn't been that long since you came running to my home and begged me to come and see what was going on with your mother. I told you that I am not a doctor, I am only a midwife, but you insisted for me to come and help her. I came and I saved your mother's life and now, you and you," she said, pointing out those that she had helped, "have the guts to come and check my house for something that you will not find, anyway? Shame on you! All of you! Go ahead and do what you have to do, if this your mission, but God is looking at you right now, making plans for you and your families, and I don't see good things coming to you. I forgive you," Maria said, making the sign of the cross in the air toward them.

Then she turned her back to them.

The Nazi team seemed to be touched by Maria's words. They looked around the yard and crossed the street number from the black list, looking ashamed. They never checked the house and they never came back.

Maria had no idea what happened behind her, but she didn't hear any door opening, so she hoped the soldiers left, leaving them alone. Maria went directly to the shed and she hugged her dog, kissing him and saying, "Thank you for saving our lives."

She took a few deep breaths and went back to the basement where everybody was waiting for her. When she opened the basement door, she could feel the surge of relief coming from downstairs and all of them started asking questions at the same time.

"Tell us what's happened outside? What was it? Who was it?"

"Nothing, our dog went crazy. Maybe he saw an animal or a bird, who knows? Our dog is an excellent dog and I love him." Their dog was a German Shepherd, beautiful and strong. Maria couldn't stop making the analogy in her mind. Ok, we have a German Shepherd dog and I had to deal with a German Nazi team! "Now, relax and pray. Things will get better; we are not alone," she told everyone there.

Titus and John came back home and everybody tried to be the first to share the events with them. John realized what his wife did, and he couldn't believe she went by herself outside to check what was happening. He was upset. "Why did you go? It could be very dangerous. There are Nazi teams going from home to home looking for Jewish people to take them as prisoners. They could arrest you."

"I know, but nothing happened. I promise to not do it again."

Later, during the night, she told her husband the truth and how it happened.

John's heart almost stopped. "No, you didn't!"

"Yes, I did it and it felt so good! I look around me and it makes me feel like a hero. But nobody has to know about this, promise!"

"I promise you, but you have to promise me you will never do it again; do not play with your life! You have our son and me; you have to live for us. What about your family that you love so much? How could you do it? Promise me again."

"I promise, you have my word," Maria said, but she knew she would do it again, as many times as necessary.

* * * *

The next day seemed to be quieter. Not as many bombs as they heard before, not so many raids. But people were afraid; certain this was only the calm before the storm. They came out of the basement, one by one, not sure if they were being watched, to be sure they were safe.

What a feeling, to see the sky above your head with no war planes dropping bombs. People had hope for a better tomorrow. They knew it was going to be hard, but they were alive. Not too many people could say that. Nora's family didn't suffer any causality, but others were not that lucky. Blocks of concrete littered the landscape, the tram's tracks were missing, and the electrical lines were gone.

Every day was bringing more difficulties, but people were determined to survive. Their church and the school next to the church were untouched. Their church, resembling a museum of paintings, was standing in full glory as a symbol of victory. So many homes had been destroyed—they were simply gone. Maria and her family realized how blessed they were to be alive. The King had been forced to leave the country, and the Russians took over, so the Germans must have lost the war. The Russian soldiers were like thieves, grabbing everything they laid their eyes on.

Maria knew how dangerous this could be, so she talked to her sister. "You have no need to go in the streets. Titus will take care of what you need and take care of Bob. I will help you with things that you cannot do or you shouldn't do. You're almost ready to bring your baby in this world. Nora, you know it won't be easy, but we are going to make it. We survived." Maria gently shook her sister's body. "We are together and this is important. We have each other."

Life was getting back to normal, slowly, one day at a time. But it was a new "normal" that everybody had to get used to. People started to feel the "Russian boot," the new normal. And nobody had ever experienced such a thing; people had no idea what exactly this was, and they knew nothing about Communism. But they could feel it wouldn't be easy. The stores were empty; the jobs gone; factories and institutions were down, not functioning, or destroyed, demolished. There was no clearer image of a country that had gone through hell.

People had to learn how to get back on their feet. A new party was formed and it was called the Communist Party. In only a few months, the party grew because almost everybody became a member. In order to keep your job, you had to be a Communist!

People had so much hate for the new regime, but they had to be quiet, not say it out loud. Ordinary or highly educated people, everybody needed safety for their families, a roof above their heads and a place to work. Saying "no" to becoming a Communist Party member, equaled being an enemy of Communism. Saying no could mean going to jail or other places where nobody would ever hear from you again. Many prominent figures, political and religious, ended up in such places, and nobody knew where they went. Fear was the word of the day, and it's a powerful word. There were times when you were afraid to talk to your friend or even a relative.

Everybody seemed to be afraid of their own shadows. It was wise to keep your thoughts for yourself, and never speak your thoughts out loud. Whispering it was a much safer way of communication.

The new regime didn't agree with religion, any kind of religion. Most of their members were people that came from villages or small towns where religion was very much respected. But they had to show they had no religious faith in order to participate in the Communist Party's actions, to show their solidarity. It was even frowned upon to have icons of the saints in your home, so people started hiding all religious items from the walls of their homes. Women stopped wearing the crosses around their necks. They had less and less money. They replaced their elegant scarves and hats with cheap things.

The war had ended, even if it didn't look like it did.

It would take time to rebuild the city, and even more time for the smiles to come back to people's faces. But there was always hope and faith. It was a hidden faith that all the people had, but they were afraid to show it. Hoping life would get better, like it was before that monstrous war.

At least, everybody hoped so.

CHAPTER THREE

Nora held her stomach and walked to her mom's house. "Mom, wake up, please! I need you to go to Maria and bring her here, fast! I am having my baby, Mom; my baby is coming, hurry up." Nora would have never dared to tell her mom to "hurry up" before, but now she had to.

Linda put something on her shoulders and ran to Maria's house. Maria had to help a neighbor the night before and it had been a difficult case. She almost couldn't do it.

Maria had to fight for both mother and the baby, but she managed to do it, saving their lives. She came home around 2:00 a.m., exhausted but happy. When she put her head on her pillow, a big smile covered her face and it took less than a minute to get to dream land.

Her mom was knocking at the door, waking everybody else but Maria. When she finally woke up, without asking any questions, she said, "Bring me some iced water," thinking of the old good times when they had ice. She realized the moment and corrected herself. "Bring me, very cold water please." She ran into the bathroom to splash some water from the faucet on her face, but it didn't do much. She needed a full bucket to pour on her head. So, she ran in the yard, grabbed the garden hose, turned it to the maximum, and let it rain down over her head and body. In few minutes, she was up and running, completely awake, ready to do her job.

Nora was in pain, but like always, she was quiet.

Titus and David went all the way to the shed, to be far away from the action, but then both of them realized that Bob was alone in the house. He was safe, of course, but they wanted to be closer to him. Peter and John were together in their home. On the way to Bob, Titus saw Maria getting ready to help her sister. He asked her if she needed his help.

Maria smiled and told Titus that this wasn't a man's job. "I know how you feel, but trust me. She will be ok; both of them will be ok. Take care of your son, Simon and my father."

Titus hugged Maria and went to be with his son.

Nora grabbed her mom's hand and held it so strong that it bruised her. She looked in Maria's eyes and said, "I trust you, I love you!"

"I know it," Maria answered, getting ready to do her job. Maria asked her mother to boil some water but she already had. Maria was thankful Linda had so much experience and she knew what was needed.

"Nora, you are doing great! A few more pushes will do it."

A small, olive-skin baby girl was born. She screamed like any other baby. Maria knew that even if the baby was small, she was healthy. She delivered so many babies that she knew it right away.

"Nora, she is so beautiful; God bless both of you."

The baby wasn't as beautiful as Peter or Bob, but for her, she was beautiful. Nora was exhausted but so happy.

Maria prepared everything, and her mom helped a lot. Maria covered the baby girl with a blanket and gave her to Nora, to hold her. What a feeling, what a joy!

Looking up, Nora said, "God, thank you, you have listened to my prayers. You have given me a boy and a girl, like I always wanted. I love you and thank you."

Maria was putting her things together, hoping she could go back to sleep, but she couldn't leave. She had to hold that precious niece in her arms, so she asked her sister to let her hold the baby for few minutes. The moment she held her, a long prayer came to Maria's mind and she made the cross sign over the baby's body, asking God to take care of that newly born baby, her niece.

"May I call her Ana?" Maria asked. "It is such a strong, beautiful name."

"Ana will be her name," Nora answered. "It is the name I wanted for my baby. Thank you for what you did for us. You should get some rest now; actually, both of us should. Mom said she would take care of everything, like she always does anyway. See you later and I cannot wait to celebrate my baby girl's birthday."

Titus and Bob were taking turns "fighting" to hold the baby. Everybody liked her name. Friends and families came to celebrate that tiny baby. Some people were coming from far away, out of town, and considering how tough the times were, it was almost a sacrifice to spend so much money when the economy was so weak, so poor. But they wanted to show their love and respect. It was a celebration of hope and love, representing the end of the war and the beginning of a new life. With the war being over, this baby girl brought the light that everybody was waiting for. They wished that Communism didn't exist, but it did.

Titus couldn't help himself from talking to everybody about his newborn baby girl. His happiness was contagious. He had a perfect family and he felt grateful for it. The only shadow over his joy was the new regime. Things were getting better, more organized. The stores seemed to be putting more goods on the shelves; people started to repair their homes with whatever they had. The city looked cleaner, and new buildings could be seen here and there. It was hard; it was a struggle, but they had hope everything would get a lot better.

Ana was growing normally, and beautiful, but Nora was concerned at how small she was. When Titus came home from his shop, she served dinner. After that, she said, "Titus, we have to do something! Ana needs more care; she is so tiny! When I take her for a walk with the stroller, people look at her and they don't know what to say, and I know they are lying when they say, 'She is so cute!' "

"Did you talk to Dr. Bitterfield? What did he say?"

Dr. Bitterfield had been their family doctor for years and years, taking care of several generations during his lifetime. Dr. Bitterfield worked for all the families in the same way Maria worked for the women in their community. He would be the one to come to for all your medical needs; you didn't need to go to his home. Even though he lived only a few minutes away from Nora's family. Babies, children, adults, Dr. Bitterfield knew them all and treated everybody with love. He was like a father to all. His doctor's suitcase looked like it had the whole world inside. Everything he needed was there, even immunizations.

"He already said there is nothing wrong with our girl, but he said we need to take her somewhere for fresh air, good quality air, and good food. The war destroyed everything. It is so hard to find the right things a new baby needs to grow healthy and normal. Her body needs more vitamins, more good nutrition. My breast milk is missing those. I hate what the war did to us, to everybody. But on the other side, on a much more positive note, Dr. Bitterfield said that Ana would become a beautiful young lady, healthy and smart. She just needs a boost!"

"Ok, I will talk to him again to see what he suggests."

After they finished dinner, Titus took Nora's hands in his and said, "I love you!"

Suddenly, Nora started crying and said, "I thought our love suffered as much as we did! Don't ask me why."

"Nothing in this world can make my love for you suffer. I live and work and exist only for you and our kids."

Nora smiled and said with a loud voice, "Tomorrow will be a better day and God will take care of us, like he always does."

* * * *

Dr. Bitterfield recommended a small mountain village close to a town where the King's palace was for the "boost" Ana needed, and it could even help Bob.

Nora remembered how the palace looked like a masterpiece. The architecture of that palace was unique, majestic and the location was friendly where people were happy to have the King stay there. The small village where Nora took her kids hadn't been touched by the war and everything was intact. The mountain village wasn't too far from the capital. Luckily, Titus had some savings for emergencies or situations like this.

They rented a beautiful cabin and started packing for the

journey. Nora tried to leave the house and things for her husband in order, and, once again, she thanked God for having such good parents and a loving family. Everybody promised to be there if Titus needed help. It was hard saying goodbye! Titus hugged his kids and kissed his wife, asking her to keep in touch and to be careful. He wanted to go with them, but he had to work; they needed the money.

Nora could not believe the view! What beauty! Huge mountains covered in snow and the small village looked like it was at the bottom of a bucket, surrounded by forests and mountains. The air was so strong that it almost made them dizzy. Clean, fresh air, exactly what Dr. Bitterfield suggested.

Nora covered Ana's face, afraid the air would be too much for the first day. What a feeling, to have too much of a good thing. She couldn't believe how people lived in this village. They were far away from the devastations of the war, far away from the bad things. These locals had no idea how lucky they were to live here. Nora stilled her racing thoughts, hired a carriage pulled by two horses—reminding her of old, good times, back in her town—and gave the address to the owner of the carriage.

Their journey had officially begun.

The cabin was breathtaking; everything was made of wood, and there were fireplaces. It was so welcoming. The owners looked like the best grandparents you could wish for. They hugged Nora and the kids, invited them to see their room, and told Nora what time dinner would be served. The first thing Nora thought of was Titus! She would be so happy to have him here, to be together in this cabin. But she knew he had to work so they could rebuild their lives, to be better for their kids' future. Ok, Nora, get real, you have a mission to accomplish, she reminded herself.

Bob was already playing. He was so smart; he could invent a toy or a game from any object he found around him.

Dinner was so delicious that it reminded Nora about the old times, the good times before the war, with happy people. She couldn't believe the fresh food! Fresh food in the middle of the winter!

Nora and Bob ate like they never ate before. The hosts were

happy to see how much Nora and Bob enjoyed the food, the house, the landscape, the air, and the atmosphere. It made them happy to see their faces. It didn't take long for Ana's cheeks to bloom with healthy color, for her to begin gaining weight.

She kept thanking Dr. Bitterfield in her mind for suggesting this amazing place. Nora was happy to see how close their cabin was to the King's palace. She hoped to be able to visit it and show Bob how beautiful the palace was.

She had invited her nephew to join them for a few days, but Maria and John weren't able to take the time off from work to bring Peter to the mountains. Nora hoped that later on, he would be able to join them for another vacation.

One day, she took her kids to visit the palace. When they arrived there, Nora asked to visit the palace, to show it to her son. She couldn't wait to see it, too.

The officer stopped them, saying they weren't allowed to go inside and the palace couldn't be visited.

"What do you mean it cannot be visited? I have visited inside with my parents."

"When?" the officer asked. "That was probably a long time ago. Now the palace belongs to the president of our country and it is an official residence. Nobody can go inside but the officials, the members of the government."

Nora was shocked, but she turned around and left, feeling frustrated. Her face was red, her eyes burning with angry tears, but she didn't want Bob to see how unhappy she was.

When they arrived back at the cabin, she ran to the kitchen where the lady of the house was and started asking non-stop questions.

The owner of the cabin thought something bad happened, because Nora's expression showed her distress.

"What's happened to the palace? They didn't let us go inside, to visit!"

"Oh, they changed the rules a long time ago. The King left the country because of the new regime. He preferred to leave the country, instead of spending the rest of his life in prison. The rules are different now. The palace is for members of the Communist Party only, and only for the big 'sharks,' you know what this means. What a waste!"

"So, I cannot show it to my son? It used to be so friendly. I remember how you could spend the whole day there, playing in the yard, looking around. What a joy. And now it is taken away from us. I remember how elegant everything was, the automobiles, the ladies, their parties. I used to go there with my parents to visit. Ok, what else will this regime take away from us? Keep smiling and be happy, it is the only thing I can say. Your husband told me that the 'new people' go to the villages surrounding the palace and fill their baskets with fresh eggs, legumes, meats from farmers' homes, without asking or paying for it. This is unheard of. They are thieves—to steal the farmers' products; they worked so hard for it. They did the same thing to my husband's shop. One day, they came inside and grabbed all the nice things and left like nothing happened. Every day, somebody comes in with a stack of applications trying to convince my husband to become a member of the Communist Party. I don't think he can refuse much longer, without complicated consequences. We heard horrible stories about men and women that refused to become members of that party."

The lady of the house replied, "I do believe it. Our neighbors have complained to the mayor about all the things those soldiers do, but he's one of them. No answers, no solutions. We have to keep our mouths shut and let the thieves take whatever they want. We are scared of these people. Actually, we are scared of everybody. You don't know any more who is who and if that person is an enemy or not. We live in terrifying times."

Nora's sadness flowed through her words. "I thought the war didn't change anything here, but it is only what you can see from the outside. The real changes aren't seen. I feel sorry for my country and for all of us. Our children have to face this horrible 'new' life. But I'm grateful we're here with you. Look at my daughter's face, how beautiful she is! Thank you for all the things you did for us. I will try to forget about the 'bad' things, like you do, and take one day at a time."

Escape

Nora waited for the kids to go to bed so she could sit down and write a letter to her husband. She wrote about the beautiful place where they were enjoying good air and fresh food. She wrote about Ana's improvements, how she looked, and how happy Bob was, playing and making friends. She wasn't sure if she should write about the conversation she had with the owner of the cabin, thinking it would be too depressing.

She convinced herself that her family had to know what was going on even in a quiet part of the country, that there were sad changes everywhere. Nora missed Titus terribly and she wished he could be here, to be together. She missed her family so much, but looking at Ana's face, her happiness replaced any other feelings. A mother will always be a mother first.

* * * *

Titus was so pleased to see his wife's handwriting on the envelope he received. He kissed it many times before opening it. He felt like they were right there, in front of him. *My God, how much I love my wife and my kids.*

After he finished reading the letter, he grabbed a piece of paper and started writing about his thoughts. He tried to say everything, saying nothing. He was tempted to write about how much people suffer, having no food and no jobs, just trying to survive.

They had to save whatever they made in order to buy the daily necessities, and his shop, with fancy things, was absolutely dead! He still thought of it as "his" shop, even if it belonged to the state now. Titus put lots of money, hard work, time and his talent into that shop and now, somebody else took it over, against his will. But to survive and be safe, you had to close your eyes and go with the flow.

Titus owed this to his family at least, he was praying to God to give him strength to continue this kind of life, but he wasn't sure about this. He tried to keep a positive tone in his letter, but knowing his wife, he knew she would be able to read in between the words. He finished the letter by promising that he would come to visit them.

As soon as he finished writing the last sentence, he realized he had to purchase a train ticket to get there. He couldn't believe this thing became an issue…a train ticket that he couldn't afford to spend money on. He had to save everything he had just for surviving.

Titus knew he didn't have another skill beyond making crystal vases and glass items, so he was very concerned about the future of his family. He was wondering what kind of job he should get, where else he could work to make money. He was really good at working with his hands, fixings things around the house that didn't work; but to get another job? His mind was working non-stop to find a solution and he finally did.

* * * *

Nora read her husband's letter and was glad to find out everybody was healthy and doing ok. After a few more weeks, she hated knowing her time in paradise was over. They belonged to their world, a world much tougher and much more difficult, so she started packing—getting ready to leave the cabin and the amazing people that opened their home and their hearts for Nora and her kids. She said goodbye to the mountains and hugged the people who treated them like they were part of their family.

She was mentally prepared to face the real world in her city, where everything you looked at had the "war stamp." She'd been born in this city; and all the people she loved and all the things she loved were here, where she belonged.

"Bob, come closer, the train is coming!"

They got on the train that took them to another world with a different future.

When they arrived at the big train station, the whole family was waiting to hug them. The hugs and kisses were endless. Titus apologized for not bringing flowers, without saying that he couldn't afford to buy them.

Nora knew this. Everybody looked poor. No hats, no high heels, no carriages, no flowers. Ok, it is what it is. We are alive and we love each other; we can make it she thought as she held her husband's hands with so much strength that it almost hurt him. "I love you."

Titus knew how much it meant to Nora to say what she just said. In all the years since they were married, Nora said these words only a couple of times. For her, the word "love" was the translation of—I would die for you, I cannot live without you, and even more. He looked in her eyes and said, "We are going to be ok, I promise."

Nora expected to hear 'I love you, too' or something similar, not what he said. She started to wonder if everything was ok. "What do you mean? Is something wrong? Is Simon all right?" It was her first thought because her father-in-law was the only one not there, so she thought maybe he was sick.

"Oh, yes," Titus answered. "My father is doing great. He cannot wait to see you and the kids. He said he wants his time with his grandchildren, but I think we have to wait a little bit longer, so Ana can play with him."

Nora believed him and she couldn't wait to get home, to their home, where love was everywhere.

The next day, Dr. Bitterfield came to see how Ana and Bob were doing. It was great to see the surprise and the satisfaction in his eyes. "I'm so glad you were able to do this for your baby girl and for Bob. Wait a minute, it seems it worked pretty well for you, too. Look at Ana's face; how healthy her skin is, the coloring is so pink. I feel like I want to kiss her cheeks, and I think I am going to do it." He bent over and kissed Ana's forehead and her cheeks. "If I asked you if you liked that small mountain village, am I right that you will answer that you would like to go back in a heartbeat? I know I'm right."

"Actually, I would love to live there forever, but I belong where my whole family is."

"I know it; we all have to face it."

"To face it, what do you mean?" Nora knew exactly what Dr. Bitterfield meant. Coming home from the train station, everywhere she looked was sadness and poverty. Her city looked dead.

"Nothing," Dr. Bitterfield answered. "We will be ok. I am so pleased with what I see looking in your kids. Do you remember when I told you that Ana would be perfect, healthy, and normal?

You were so concerned about her weight, and look at her now."

"I do remember it, but it seems almost impossible to feed them the same way I did it in the mountains."

"I know. We all have this problem. The farmers used to bring fresh eggs, milk, sour cream, chickens, and all the fresh food, but they stopped coming. They don't have enough for themselves. Nora, you are a strong, young woman. Remember that everybody and everything depends on you. Men are strong, but in a different way."

"Yes, I will do whatever it takes to protect my family," Nora said, smiling.

"Nora, I forgot to mention one more thing. This is the last time I'll able to come and check on your kids in your home. They gave me permission to let all my patients know that from now on, they have to come and see me at the new clinic."

"What clinic? What's happened; why do we have to bring our kids to the clinic; what's wrong with our home?" Nora asked question after question. "Who is 'they'?"

"The new regime, the Communist Party, and the new government. Last month, my practice was confiscated and I was given a job at this clinic that I told you about. I will be paid a low salary, but at least I can bring all of you there. It is so new that I have no idea how things will work. This is something new for the government too, so it will take time to figure out payments, working with employees, creating unions, and getting organized. I thank God, I am old enough that I don't have to see all of these changes, but I feel really sorry for the young generations. What times we live in, what we have to deal with. I will schedule Ana's next appointment, so she can get all her immunizations in order. Ok, now I have to leave, but not before kissing you and the kids. I love you, and I will see you soon at the clinic; this is the address." Dr. Bitterfield handed her a handwritten note with the name and the address, saying there was no phone yet, so Nora would have to come and check the place first, before bringing the kids. He hugged Titus and shook his hand vigorously.

* * * *

When Dr. Bitterfield was talking about his medical practice being confiscated, Titus remembered that not long ago a team of Communist workers entered his shop and told him to start making an inventory list with absolutely everything on the shelves and in the closets.

"Why do you need 'my inventory?" Titus had asked with a livid face.

"Because this shop will belong to the Department of Internal Commerce and whoever is the owner, or owners will become our employees and work for us."

"Leave the shop now, or I will hurt you bad, really bad. Go now." He opened the door.

One by one, the workers left but not without a warning, "We are leaving now, but we'll be back with a new lock and papers for you to sign."

Titus had felt so angry that he wanted to break everything he'd made with his hands, but an image of Nora surrounded by their kids came to his mind, so he calmed down and tried to forget about it, but he knew the clock was ticking. He never told Nora about the horrible incident and he realized, after listening to Dr. Bitterfield, that it was the perfect moment to talk to his wife about the future of their shop.

Titus sat down on a chair and asked Nora to join him.

She looked at him smiling, thinking he wanted to talk about what they just heard from Dr. Bitterfield. Nora sat on a chair and said, "Can you believe it, poor Dr. Bitterfield! He is like a father for all of us, for the whole family. But we have to do what he said and go to the clinic. At least we are going to have the same doctor. It is so important for our kids, especially since they're so used to him."

"I know," Titus said, "I like him too. Everything he does for our kids and for us is perfect and he puts all his heart into what he does. He is a jewel." He waited a moment before he continued, "Nora, I have something to tell you that I wanted to tell you a long time ago, but I waited for you to come home."

"What? Is it about Dr. Bitterfield?" Nora asked.

"No, it is about me."

"Are you sick? What's happened?"

"No, thank God! I am fine, but things have changed."

"What has changed? Do you mean the things between us?" Nora asked.

"No, this has nothing to do with me and you as a couple. It is about our shop."

"What about the shop? Did it catch fire?"

"No. Nora, I have to give up the shop. This time it is serious. They tried before, but now it is real; it will happen soon."

"Give up for what, to whom? Do you owe money to somebody?"

"No, it is about the new regime. There will be no more private properties; everything will belong to the state. The state is the employer now, and we will be its employees. Like Dr. Bitterfield mentioned, we will be paid a minimal salary to survive. It will be very hard to work in 'your place' when it is not yours anymore. In one of the letters I got from them, and I did receive quite a few, it said that I should feel honored to be one of the state employees!"

"Say no. What is so hard?" Nora said.

"Oh, you don't get it, Nora. That is not an option. They will come soon, close the doors, change the locks, do their own inventory, change the name of the shop, and bring new people to work there if I refuse to work for them. They can throw me in jail if I refuse to work for them; it isn't a joke. Nora, we live in a much different world, and I'm not happy, not at all."

"Titus, I will get a job and help with money. My mom can watch the kids, thank God; she is still strong and healthy." Nora gazed at her husband, lifted his chin up, and continued, "I thought I would be shocked to hear one bad thing after another one, but I am getting used to it with all these 'new things.' We will be ok; I know it. Don't be upset, we'll make it. Let's take care of the kids; they have to go to bed. Tomorrow is another day! We have each other and somebody above is watching us, helping us. I love you."

* * * *

Escape

The next day, Titus went to work at the shop and Nora tried to cook his favorite food, to make him worry less and be happier. She looked in the pantry and said, "How can I cook, when there is nothing in the pantry? Let me see what Maria or my mom has, so I can put something together."

Everybody's pantry was the same—empty. The whole family put together whatever money they had and bought some groceries and produce to be able to cook some food. There had never been such a problem, food! It was ridiculous. Maria was the only one bringing home some good stuff, but only once in a while. She asked her patients to pay her in food rather than money. The Jewish families were doing much better by having their own government. It was called The Jewish Federation and they were getting international help. It was like a state in a state. Getting help from all over the world, their Jewish friends were doing a lot better than the rest of the population. After a couple of months, Maria's husband John got more work fixing watches and jewelry.

Maria got a job in a hospital, and they were bringing home necessary things for the whole family to use.

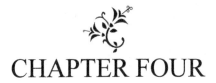

CHAPTER FOUR

Titus was still in shock. He was still thinking of those days when the Russian soldiers came to his shop and grabbed everything they could carry in their arms. The image of his old father witnessing this kind of robbery haunted him. He almost had a heart attack when that happened. So, Titus asked his father not to come to the shop anymore to help, because he wasn't sure what the next day could bring. The Russian boot was everywhere, now followed by those turned into Communists.

You go with it or you could say goodbye to your life and die proud! It became a motto of the new lifestyle.

Of course, I have to become a member of the Communist Party, to save what I love the most: my family. How can I look in their eyes knowing that I didn't do what I could have done to protect them?

His inner voice answered, "Do you call this protection? No, it is called 'shame.' How can you do such a horrible thing, to become a tool of oppression, an instrument of destruction?"

Titus continued the dialogue, "You are right, but can you see your friends? They made the pact with the evil, becoming members of the Party, and now they are doing a lot better than you and your family and even their children are treated differently in school. I can keep going with examples around you, but I know for sure you already know I'm right. I refuse to admit it, I see so many of my friends losing their conscience and pride, looking like they have been brainwashed, only to have a 'better' life. Good for them, but I cannot do it."

Titus's monologue made him decide his future.

Escape

* * * *

Ana was almost three years old when her aunt Maria gave birth to a handsome baby boy. Nora helped her as much as she could and so did their mother, but they had to call a midwife to be sure everything was done well and finish things. When Nora was holding the newborn in her arms, her maternal feelings bloomed. She wanted a new baby too! For a moment, she forgot about the times she was living in. For one minute, she forgot how difficult it was to survive, to raise a family, to feed and take care of your children.

She looked at Maria with love and gave her the baby, her baby, to hold him. "Congratulations, God bless both of you and all our family. He was born in love; I love Peter, your older son, but this handsome boy is going to be my favorite nephew. Do you still want to call him Chris? I love this name; it is so close to Jesus," Nora said. "Everybody will know he is a Christian, without even asking!"

"Do you think it is a good thing nowadays, to be a Christian?" Maria asked.

"Not at this moment, but the good times will come and his name will be just perfect. Christi, Christian, Chris." Nora played with the baby's name. She liked the way it sounded and she kept saying the newborn baby's name, to choose which one she liked the most.

"Isn't this sad that you want a beautiful name for your newborn baby boy, but you are scared it could be politically incorrect?" Maria exclaimed, saying exactly what she was thinking.

"What a world we live in! Do not worry, please," Nora said, "call him the name you want. He is your son. You have the right to do so."

"Nobody has rights anymore; we have only duties."

"You are perfectly right, forget about it. Get some rest, you look exhausted."

"I am grateful I was able to have an easy delivery. The midwife helped me a lot. Maybe I will work with her in the future."

"Are you crazy? It hasn't even been an hour since you gave birth and your mind wonders about work already!"

"Nora, life goes on," Maria answered almost sleeping. Her

eyelids were getting heavier and soon she fell in a deep sleep.

Nora and her mom were taking turns holding the baby; they didn't want to put him down.

Peter, the brand new big brother, came closer and started complaining, "He is my brother. I am old enough to raise him. I know how." Peter was a really smart child. His curiosity for the human body made his parents think that he might become a doctor.

Maria could see herself in him. He was trying to help everybody, anywhere, anytime. "You're right, Peter. You are his older brother and you will help your parents to raise Chris."

"I like his name and I like the way he looks. His eyes look like Japanese eyes," he said.

"What did you just say? What do you know about Japanese people? Did you read about Japanese eyes? Where did you come up with this? You are funny!" Nora said to her nephew.

"Don't you see his eyes are almost closed?"

"You're right; his eyes look like you said. But in a few months, Chris's eyes will be like yours. You are brothers and you will look alike."

When Nora let Peter hold his baby brother for the first time, he was almost shaking. Nora's hands were underneath the baby to be sure he was safe.

Ana couldn't take her eyes away from her new cousin. It was the first time she saw a newborn baby.

Bob was waiting for his turn to hold the baby. Bob was almost five years old but looked and behaved more maturely than other kids his age.

Nora looked at them and a warm feeling enveloped her. She thought... this is happiness; this is the reason we exist. Nothing compares with this image; I want to keep them safe and healthy. She felt like she had four children, not only two. Nora knew her sister had the same feelings. They were good mothers and those four cousins would love each other like brothers; they would grow together as brothers and sister. What a blessing. She sent out a little prayer: "God, protect them, keep them healthy, and I will do everything you want me to do. Then she kissed them, one by one, and let the big ones go to their grandmother to be spoiled.

The kids adored their grandparents, especially their grandmother. Everything she did for them, they liked it; her food, and her cookies especially, were delicious.

Nora spent time holding Chris, waiting for Maria to wake up and feed the baby. The baby's face was smiling and Nora was so happy to look at him and wonder at what was in his mind that made him smile.

* * * *

After a few days, Maria took her children to be seen by Dr. Bitterfield at the new clinic. The clinic was clean, and Dr. Bitterfield seemed to like his new place. He checked the kids and gave Maria an excellent health report for her children.

Considering how hard it was to have good, fresh food, this was like a gift from God, to know her doctor was satisfied with the results, measurements, weight, and all the other things tested in the check-up of her kids. "Thank you, Doctor, you made my day brighter. My family will be happy to hear all the good news. When is my sister bringing her children? Should I ask the nurse?"

"No, I have no nurse now, maybe in the future. I have to handle everything alone. I'm ok. The only good thing about working in a clinic is that I have a schedule, not like before. I'm not allowed to see patients after work hours. There is another department dealing with the after-hours situations. I make no money, but I have more time now and it is ok, because I am getting older. My wife is very happy, and she puts me to work around the house."

Maria and Dr. Bitterfield hugged each other and the kids kissed the doctor's cheeks. They loved him like they loved their grandfather. Peter and his cousins never cried when they went for a check-up or immunizations. What a doctor!

Maria came home and announced the good news to everybody, spreading happiness around her.

* * * *

Nora knew it was her turn to take the kids to be seen by their doctor. So, Nora waited a few more days and when the appointment day arrived, she went with her children to the new clinic. She'd been there before and she liked the place. Of course, it had been much better to have the doctor coming to your home than having to go there with two kids, but this was the new rule.

Nora was happy too. Dr. Bitterfield was very pleased with the way Ana was growing, being as tall as other girls her age. She had made up the difference. Her weight was normal and she'd started to look really cute, not like when she was a baby.

Bob looked like he enjoyed playing sports. He was tall and strong, and moved around very quickly. His love for soccer made him move that fast. He loved playing chess also. Soccer and chess, two things that don't go hand in hand usually, but for some reason they worked wonderfully in Bob's case.

Nora and her children came back home and the whole house and their big yard was full of laughter, joy, and happiness.

The children loved going to school, except Chris. Bob, Peter, and Ana had good grades, and all of them loved reading. Chris was very smart and he had his own world. Going to school was something he didn't enjoy, but he had his own way of learning things.

* * * *

Time went by and Maria and Nora were surrounded by their children and husbands. Peter and Chris were always happy to be close to their mom, to be spoiled by her. Maria was spoiling her children more than Nora, but it seemed the kids didn't care much. She was spoiling them in a different way and they adored her. Sometimes, Nora's children wished to be kissed as much as their cousins were by Maria, but Bob and Ana knew that their mother was stricter than their aunt.

Peter, the oldest of them all, was the boss, he was the leader. The cousins knew where to ask for help when they needed help.

Peter was the answer, and he was extremely happy to offer help; he loved being the older cousin. Peter knew that the word "cousin" wasn't the right one; they were brothers and they would always be brothers.

The country was in "recovery" mode. The new regime imposed its new rules, tough rules that everybody had to obey. It seemed unreal, but people learned fast how to fake their love for the Communist Party. There were meetings all over the country, parades to show love for the new regime, for the leader of the Party.

They were taking people from their work places and telling them to go and stand along the large boulevard where the leader of the country would show up to receive applause and flowers. Nobody could say no. You could, but the next day you would have no job to go to.

The young people, who didn't know as much as the older ones knew, were enjoying those parades, loving the free time!

Ana was almost old enough to start elementary school. She couldn't wait to go to school. Living right across the street, Ana was familiar with all the school activities; she could see the children coming in the morning, playing in the schoolyard during the breaks, and then leaving the school. She already felt like she'd been there forever. The teachers could see Ana's home and her yard, and this didn't seem to bother Ana, Bob, Peter, or Chris. If it did bother Chris, he didn't show it.

Once Ana began school, Nora would check her homework daily to be sure she was doing it right. It wasn't necessary, though, because Ana was a really good student. But for Nora, checking it was a mother thing. Bob liked to be her mentor too, being patient and trying to teach his sister more about mathematics.

Nora realized how many "Communist ideologies" were popping up every day in her children's homework assignments, which she didn't agree with, but she couldn't say one word about it. Her hands were tied.

Nora had to keep her mouth shut; she had to learn what the new regime wanted the students to learn. She was so upset to see how the Communist regime forced the whole country to become atheists.

The religion classes had been eliminated from all schools, all over the country, including colleges, universities, and any other form of education.

People became afraid to go to church, to have icons on the walls of their homes, to have religious items, or even to keep a Bible in the house. You never knew who could "visit" your home or if your home was on the list of the houses that had to be checked.

People learned how to play safe. It was so sad to see all this going on around you.

One day, Nora said to her daughter, "You always have to try to do the right things, to be a good person and help as much as you can, so God can see what a good human being you are, even if he knows everything we do."

Ana was quiet and listening to her mother when suddenly she said, "What God? Who is God? My teacher told us there is no God and that we're not allowed to mention this word or to make the cross sign, like you told me to do. She also said that we aren't allowed to pray or to read any book talking about God. Mom, I don't like what she's telling us, but she told us that we will be punished and that we will be hit with a wooden stick if we ever do it. Mom, I don't believe her; I believe you."

Nora's eyes were full of tears when she hugged her daughter and her son. The kids' eyes were very sad. Nora's heart was full of sadness and anger. What those people do to innocent minds, pure hearts!

She needed to keep calm and not show her children her anger and her sadness, so she kissed them and, with a loving voice, she told them, "Later on, both of you will understand how things are. You're so right; we live in a world where things aren't what they used to be. It's hard for you to listen to two different voices, one at home and one at school. Both of you are my children that I love more than anything in this world, but never forget that you are Christian human beings and God loves you, both of you. Keep this in your heart and don't talk to anybody about what we talk at home. Ana, you are so young now, but the time will come when you will understand what your mother is trying to tell you. The day will come, but till then, don't talk to anybody about this subject, please."

"I won't talk to anybody, but can I talk to my cousins?"

"Of course," Nora said. "They're like brothers to you. They are your family. I know how much you love all of them. They adore you too."

CHAPTER FIVE

Month after month went by, and Titus was going to work every day, but his heart was broken. His face often revealed the sadness he had in his heart; even when he made huge efforts to hide it.

His love for his family was the only reason he kept going to a place where he felt miserable. He hated each second of his work time, and he was happy only when he was home with his wife and children.

Bob and Ana jumped on his neck every time he came home. What a joy! The moment he walked into his home, it was like sunshine all over, hugs, kisses, laughter, and love.

Titus started talking to his inner voice again.

How can I be so sad when I have these two amazing children that love me so much? And how can I be so sad when Nora is the love of my life? How many people have what I have? I try not to think about what happened with my shop and the new situation and try to get used to working for the state, but maybe I'm a lot weaker than other men. I have tried, I tried! So why do I have those dark gray clouds in my heart and in my mind? What's wrong with me? Am I a coward? Am I that weak? Why can't I adapt to what everybody already has? Why do I have to be different? How can I dare to resist all these changes when the whole country has already kneeled? Look around you, wake up, and take care of your children's future. It is not their fault they were born under such circumstances. You aren't the only one affected by Communism; you just have to become one of them and go ahead with your life.

Escape

When he got to work, he checked a few drawers that were typically untouched by the new workers, finding photos and small items that brought nice memories to his mind, making him smile.

He pulled all the photos from the walls, wondering why the new boss didn't do it, and he put them in a suitcase. Among his other things, Titus found some savings that he'd forgotten about; not much, but enough for a thought to bloom in his mind. When the time came to go home, Titus looked around his shop, locked the door, and said to himself, "I will be back, or maybe not; I will think about coming back. But, only God knows if I will be back."

On the way home, he stopped to exchange a few words with one of his old friends, Andrew, that worked for a travel agency. He wondered how it was possible for his friend to make a living when so many people barely had money to provide food for their families, forget about traveling. But Titus forgot about the new class of the population, the new kind of people who could afford to travel. The new Communists, the members of the leader's party, they had money to go abroad, to visit places, and to deposit secret funds in Switzerland or other safe places. These kinds of people had learned quickly how to take advantage of the new power.

Titus knocked at the door, and Andrew opened it, clearly surprised to see his friend standing in front of his door. "Oh my God, Titus, how are you doing? Come inside, I'm so glad to see you. I cannot believe you stopped by."

Titus followed his friend inside the house and was invited to take a seat.

Andrew offered him a glass of water, pulled up a chair, and sat next to Titus. His old friend looked so surprised, Titus wondered if he had become a ghost!

"So, how are you? Why have you stopped to see me? I still remember the good times we spent together, free of worries, when we had no idea what freedom meant. Now we know and what a price we pay. Ok, tell me what I can do for you?"

Without too much of an introduction, Titus asked his friend if he still worked for the same travel agency that he used to, because he wanted to ask him a question.

"Yes, I do, but now the business is run by different people. I don't like them, but I have to work to bring some money home. And I love what I do because I make people happy."

"Ok, if you are still there, I want you to check the availability for one night at the small palace located in the mountains. I remember there is a pavilion for parties, for guests," Titus said. "Is it still there, or have they changed the rules even there?"

"What did you say? The castle? Do you have that much money? Are you insane? None of us have ever spent a night in that place. It's magnificent and outrageously expensive. You have to be joking, are you?"

"No, I'm not joking, I am very serious about spending a night with my wife and a few family members."

"Oh my God, you must be rich. I'm glad; I'll get my commission!"

"Not only will you get your commission, but you and your wife are invited too," Titus said. "And I'm not rich, but I have some savings and I always dreamed about going there. Call me as soon as you get the details about this, please."

"Are you kidding me? I work in the travel industry and I've never been to that place," Titus's friend kept saying. He couldn't believe what just happened to him. He thought Titus had to be mentally sick or he had another source of money.

"Now you can go to that palace. I'm glad you were home so we could put this project together. I have to leave now, and I'll wait for your call."

"Do you have a certain date in mind? Are you celebrating a special event? Is this your wedding anniversary?" he insisted, wanting to find out what all this was about. Without getting a response, Andrew continued, "Ok, I will start working on this right away. I only need a deposit from you."

Titus gave his friend a deposit and left. His mind was galloping, trying to invent something to justify the money for Nora. When he arrived home, the happiness surrounded him from everywhere, but his mind raced. What a coward I am; I don't deserve what I have. How many times have I said this to myself and still… It's the right thing to do.

* * * *

The next day, Titus worked hard trying to prepare a document to show his wife. He knew exactly all the questions Nora would ask. It took him a few days to get it done. The day he was satisfied with the results of his falsification, he went home. The first thing he told Nora was, "We are going to spend a weekend at Bran castle, in the guests' pavilion. So, you can start packing. We're going to enjoy each second spent there. I cannot wait to be together."

"What did you say? Who has money for the castle? What is wrong with you? Why do you joke like this, Titus?"

"I have the money, and we're going there for a weekend."

"Did you steal money from somebody?"

"How could you think that way? Have I have ever stolen money or anything else? Do you remember me doing things like this?"

"No, but how do you have money? Who gave it to you? What did you do to get that kind of money?"

"Nora, I have been compensated for the shop. The government paid me a small amount of money for taking the shop away from me."

"This cannot be true. We know so many people in our situation and nobody, I mean, nobody, got compensated for what was taken away from them. This regime doesn't do business like that. You're lying to me! Tell me where the money came from."

"If I show you the papers, are you going to believe me?" Titus said.

"Show me the document." She was so angry, she didn't even say please.

Titus knew how to answer all her questions; he had an answer for everything. He handed her a paper that looked real.

Nora grabbed it and she read it few times, still not believing her husband. "Even as I hold this paper in my hands, I still don't believe you. Why should they pay you and nobody else?"

"I got lucky," Titus answered with a smile.

"No, this is a fake document," Nora said.

"Why don't you look in the light and see the government stamp? I couldn't fake this. Can't you see the seal? Nora, believe me, I was lucky to be compensated for the shop."

"No, absolutely no. I don't believe it. Let's say it is true, why should we spend money going to a place when we don't have to go? Why spend the money when life is so hard and we don't have enough for food, uniforms, taxes, and so many other things? We should save it for the future, for our kids' future. I really don't understand what is going on in your mind. I never saw you like this. Something is wrong with you, and 'm ready to sit down and listen to you, to figure out what's in your mind. Titus, I love you, but what you're trying to do right now, it's more than my mind can take. You have to explain it to me."

"The only thing I ask of you is to let me have this party Nora!"

"You never liked to leave the house. You never liked parties, and now you ask for one? I just don't get it. I don't get it," she answered.

"You will, you will. I know it," Titus said with a soft voice.

Nora stared at her husband's face trying to solve this puzzle. "Titus, it's so hard to read you now. I'm very upset because of what you want to do. I can't understand you. Something is going on. Please, open your heart like you always did; tell me what is bothering you. Let's put our minds together and do the best we can for our family. Did you forget about Ana and Bob?"

"Nora, I have nothing to hide from you. I love you and our kids more than words can say. Let me have this party; it will be my way to say goodbye to the old times and to say hello to the new life. I need an outlet for my heart."

"We aren't the only ones going through these kinds of things. We have to adjust to it, and do our best. I know it is hard, but we have to try."

"Some people can do it. Some can adjust to the new life, or they pretend they do, but some like me can't! For my family's sake, I will try hard to adapt to their rules and I will try harder to be happy, like I used to be before."

"I'm glad to hear you say this. I'm sorry but there is no other way," Nora said.

"Yes, there is—yes, there is!" Titus whispered with a low voice, looking deep into his wife's eyes.

"I can't believe I am saying this…but if this party means so much to you, even if I don't understand your reason, let's have it. I'll go with you for the weekend and I will ask my parents to take care of our children," Nora said sadly

* * * *

The winter was heavy and the record-setting snowfall left a thick covering on the roofs of the houses. The kids were playing on the roofs. In this kind of weather, there would be no trams, no electric trolleys. People worked hard, shoveling to create the room for going to work or buying food, all the necessary activities of daily life.

Deep down, Nora could only think of this "party" as a waste of the money that they were in so much need of… the entire family. She couldn't stop thinking that something strange had happened to her husband.

She'd been thinking about Titus's strange behavior and realized she might not have paid attention to some of Titus's words. Why, he had said 'yes, there is!' Did he know something she didn't? Maybe it was his way of promising he would be ready to start a new life and try to be happier. *I'm sure this is what he tried to tell me, I am sure.* For now, she felt exhausted and knew tomorrow would be another hard day.

She talked to God in her own way, like she always did and thanked him for everything, but tonight, she added a new prayer, "God, please help Titus to see the right path, light his way and his mind, and let him become the man he used to be, happy. God, my husband is not happy and his mind is tormented; he needs your peace, give it to him, God, please. I love you."

Titus was sleeping already. Nora gazed at her handsome husband and realized how calm his face looked. She loved seeing his face so calm and relaxed. He had an enigmatic smile she might call it relief, on his face. She paused at this. Why does he look like this? Just because of the party? It makes no sense.

You are too tired and your mind imagines things that don't exist. You better go to bed and sleep. Tomorrow you will need all the energy that you are wasting now.

* * * *

Andrew couldn't believe how lucky he was to be asked to plan everything for his dear friend Titus, and on top of this, to be invited to the party! He tried to explain it to his wife, Lara. "You know I thought Titus, you know him, my friend was a normal person. A successful businessman, a very intelligent person, but after the conversation I had with him today, I changed my mind."

"What do you mean? What happened? Is he sick?" Lara asked.

"I cannot say if it is something wrong with him, but for some reason, I think my friend has lost his mind!"

"Why? He's such a nice gentleman. I admire him and his family. They're a model for me," she stated.

"You see, that's why! How somebody like Titus can spend the last penny on a party nowadays, when everybody struggles to survive? A normal person wouldn't do it."

Lara was shocked. "What party? Are they going to have a party? With what money?"

Andrew sat down with his wife and told her the whole conversation he had with Titus. His wife's eyes were getting bigger and bigger and he could see how shocked she was.

She spoke slowly, "So many people have lost their minds after the Communists came, but I never thought Titus would be one of them! He seemed to be so down to earth, so calm, so contented. I kind of envied his wife for being so lucky to have such a husband."

Andrew pretended to not hear his wife's last sentence, her words about Titus. It made him jealous, but he didn't have time to argue, and he knew she was right. Titus was such a gentleman, a good father, and an excellent husband.

Escape

* * * *

Titus received a phone call from Andrew, telling him that everything was taken care of, the rooms and the party. The only thing Titus had to do is buy the train tickets.

It was so unusual to have a party with so many guests, to celebrate and have a good time. What an event! Nora's parents gladly accepted the invitation to take care of the kids, and they tried hard to not ask questions.

Maria and her husband were the same way: trying to let things go their way and hoping to find out later on what the real reason was for the party—why Titus wanted to spend a fortune on a party?

There were too many questions. "Let's get ready and have fun": this was the main thing in people's minds. Many years had passed since the word 'party' had even been a part of their vocabulary. Many, many years ago...

Nora packed few things that she hadn't touched for years, fancy earrings and nice jewelry. She never thought she would ever wear them again. It seemed so strange to dress like this when people around her suffered.

Titus invited a few couples that were close to them. They were very good people with high education and moral values. These people also couldn't believe that he'd invited them to go to the mountains and have a party. They assumed it was something extremely important for Titus and his wife to spend so much money when the times were so hard, but they accepted the invitation. Even though buying the train ticket was a financial effort for almost everybody invited.

When the day came, Nora and her husband hugged their kids like never before, especially Titus. His eyes were full of tears and he couldn't let the kids go from his arms. He kissed them with so much love that it almost hurt them.

Nora had to pull him away from the kids to avoid being late at the train station.

The trip was unbelievable. It was snowing hard, and they could see huge mountains of snow. They were lucky the train was still running.

When they arrived at their destination, the sight was breathtaking; the castle was illuminated like a fairytale. It looked like they had arrived in a different world. It was the first time Titus felt grateful to the new regime—for keeping this part of the castle opened—even if it was so, they could make more money. It was an amazing view.

Nora thought about when she and their kids had arrived not too far from here and how happy they were there. The snow looked like a fluffy blanket, covering everything in white. The lights reflected in the snow shining like an invitation to the show of lights.

Everybody was mesmerized. Nobody said one word. The beauty surrounding them was more than they could ever dream of. The castle looked like the ones you only saw in your dreams. The slats pulled by strong white horses took the guests to the pavilion, where hot baths were waiting for them. The waiters were waiting with hot drinks, and everybody was treated like royalty.

After resting and getting used to their rooms, the guests arrived. Each of the couples looking elegant and radiant. What a party! The ballroom was illuminated and magnificent, but for most of them, Nora included, a little bit intimidating. What a splendor; you usually see this only once in a lifetime.

Were the same thoughts on everybody's minds? Did they think: What a contrast, what a difference between where they came from and where they were now? Nora wasn't as happy as she thought she would be. She knew it would be one night only, one day only, and after that, they would go back to the other world, the world where she belonged, the world where her children lived, where her family was. But she wouldn't let those thoughts spoil the moment.

"Enjoy now when you can," she said to herself as she tried to put all these thoughts behind her and take advantage of the moment. She danced all night with the love of her life; she kissed him with passion and love. Everybody was having fun; their faces were full of joy. Nora found herself thanking God for this time she had with her husband. Food and drinks were everywhere. The couples were covering the dance floor with happy steps. Nora's feelings were confused; she could sense something wasn't right. She couldn't say what exactly it was, but her instincts were telling her to be aware.

To be aware of what? she asked herself, looking in the mirror in their fabulous room. What is wrong with you, girl? Get your mind together. This is what Titus wanted, just do it. He has never asked you to do something like this before. Let him have what he wants. Go and get a drink and some good food and live the moment, feel better. Then in a few minutes, her mind started up again with the doubts. You know your intuition is trying to tell you something, you know you're right to feel so unsettled about this, but what can you do? Nothing. So, go dance and enjoy the party. Put your happy smile on your pretty face and play the game your husband wants you to play. Fool yourself, Nora; be happy for a night.

Titus was smiling, toasting, dancing and making everybody feel welcome and special. He treated all his guests like queens and kings. He thanked everybody for accepting his invitation and let them know how much they meant to him and his wife.

Nora was getting tired and she asked Titus if he was ready to go to bed.

* * * *

"I will be there in a minute," Titus told her. "I just have to be sure everybody is situated and taken care of. I won't stay long, wait for me." He kissed his wife deeply and sweetly then left to finish the things he had to. He said goodbye to everybody and tipped the waiters generously then asked one of the waiters to bring a slat closer. He asked to be taken to the train station.

The waiter did what he was asked to, but his eyes were wide open like an unanswered question.

Titus avoided the scene, grabbed his winter coat, and ran through the door. Once on the slat, he covered himself with the thick white blanket and looked back at the bedroom windows, where the love of his life was sleeping, or maybe she was still waiting for him. Tears, sadness, mixed feelings, memories were running through his mind, but nothing could stop him from finishing his plan, because he did have a plan!

His family would get a decent amount of money they could live on, until they found a better way to survive; hopefully, the times would change.

The snow looked so white you could see everything around. He got in the train and he said an imaginary goodbye to his beautiful wife. He waited about a half an hour after the train started moving, gaining more speed, to be sure nobody could rescue him.

Titus opened the door of the train car and he threw himself into death's arms.

* * * *

Nora woke up, pulled back the elegant curtains, and let the light come in. She suddenly realized that Titus never came back to the room. She thought that maybe, he woke up earlier and was waiting for her with a hot coffee and nice breakfast. So, happy and singing, she took a long, hot shower, got dressed to take a slat ride with her love, and went down the stairs into the lobby where guests were enjoying their breakfast. She greeted everybody with a smiling face and started looking for Titus, asking if anyone knew where her husband was. No one knew the answer.

Nobody had seen him since last night. Nora was angry and felt uncomfortable. What about an affair? She thought, and her mind kept racing: Of course, it was an affair. This is the reason he didn't come back to the bedroom. The reason he'd been acting so strange. Could he be sleeping with another woman? She shook her head; she knew better. This couldn't be real. Her husband adored her; he would never behave that way. Nora knew her husband wasn't like that.

She knew she needed to stop thinking that way and look for him, so they could go back home. Forgetting about breakfast, she needed to find Titus. Her friends checked all the rooms and asked around about Titus; no answers.

The waiter that helped Titus with the slat left right after the party was over. He was the only one that knew Titus left in the middle of the night.

CHAPTER SIX

Nora had to pack and leave; her kids were waiting for them to come back home.

She said goodbye and got in the train, hoping that Titus got home before her.

When she arrived home, she kissed her children and her family members and asked about Titus. She tried to ask those questions when the kids weren't there, but everybody was asking about Titus already. Where was he?

Nora had the same questions to ask, with no answers. The kids were too young to realize why, but not too young to realize something wasn't normal, and looking at their faces, you could see how puzzled they were.

Nora was surrounded by all of her family, looking concerned and sad, when the phone rang.

"Mrs. Nora Salomea?" a voice asked at the other end.

"Yes, this is she."

"Hello. This is the railroad station police department, and I am so sorry to inform you that your husband has had a fatal accident after falling from the train. He was pronounced dead at the scene. I'm so sorry, my condolences."

"What? This is impossible. It couldn't be him!"

"Is his name Titus? We have a potential address, as well." He started listing the numbers of her address.

"Oh my God, oh my God," Nora said, dropping the phone. "He's dead; my husband is dead." Just a second later, she fainted.

John reached out to catch her from her falling.

The kids rushed to her, scared and screaming. "Grandma, grandpa, come quickly; fast, fast!"

"What is going on?" They saw Nora lying down on the floor and Maria trying to shake her.

"Nora, wake up, please, wake up!"

Nora opened her eyes and instantly remembered what she'd just learned—her husband was dead! She hugged her kids, her mom, and her sister and for a few minutes, she couldn't say one word. Tears rolled down on her and her kids' faces. They were quiet and scared.

Ana had no idea why her mom was crying, but Bob realized they didn't have a father anymore. At ten years old, his life has changed forever. He ran outside and washed his face with snow, crying and calling his father back. When he came back in the room, his sister was holding their mom's hands and crying because her mom and everybody in the room were crying. She looked so scared, trying to understand what happened, why her mom was crying, and where her father was.

Titus's father was devastated. What a tragedy! Simon looked lost and his expression was livid. He tried to help his daughter-in-law and stay with his grandchildren as much as possible, so the women could do the necessary things for his son's burial.

No parent should go through this; no parent should lose a child. It is against nature. Dark thoughts crowded his brain. Why, God, why? My son had the best he could have for the times we live in, an amazing wife and two healthy, beautiful children—a wonderful family! Why didn't you take me?

* * * *

Nora brought her husband's remains home and had a modest funeral celebrating and honoring his life. The whole community was present, supporting the family. The priest performed one of the most impressive ceremonies that he ever did. Tears were flooding all over the cemetery. People didn't feel the cold, didn't care about the big snow; their hearts have been so touched by looking at the family that lost their father and husband. The whole community looked at those children that needed their father more than anything, to be protected and to grow in a safe, loving family. What a tragedy! Why did he want to have that party so much; what was the secret? There were questions on everybody's minds; something must have happened there.

Nora was so absent mentally, she almost didn't know where she was. She looked like she had no idea her husband was dead. Her mother gave her some tea to drink and added a few drops of a special elixir that takes your mind away for a few hours. Thank God, she did because then Nora could be unconscious for the whole ceremony. But Nora's elixir ran out and she remembered the situation. She started screaming and she wanted to throw herself over the edge.

Her sister and John pulled her back, holding her tight.

Bob and Ana were wrapped around their mom's body, without letting her move. She was surrounded by life and love. They were pulling her back to life. The only thing she could say was, "Why? Why? I love you; our kids need you. Why? Why?"

The burial plot that belonged to their family for centuries was located in the heart of the city, which had developed around the cemetery. Superstitions and the fear of ghosts were the only reasons the Communists didn't destroy the cemetery to build their ugly buildings.

The family came home from the cemetery, and Nora's mother prepared some food for people to eat and put some wine on the table. It was a custom for people to eat and drink some wine after a burial.

Nora and her children were in another room, holding their hands together. Maria was watching over them. She couldn't keep her tears from washing her beautiful face. She promised to herself to take care of her sister and her nephews, as if they were her own family. They were like a family but now it would be so different.

I have a new responsibility as an older sister. Why did he have to die, God, tell me why? Maria thought. He was so young. Now his children will suffer so much, why? What was wrong in his mind? Why did he want that party? I will never understand why. Nobody pays for a party when you struggle to put food on the table!

Maria started praying now. "God, show me the reason; there had to be a reason. I never heard about a situation like this! My sister is so young and now she has to raise two children on her own. I will help her all my life. Whatever I have, she will have." Maria made this promise to herself.

* * * *

In the months following Titus's death, Linda helped a lot with things around the house to give Nora time to mourn her husband. One day, Nora and her mother were sitting in the yard, knitting and talking.

"I will take care of the house, but you have to take care of your children's future and yours too!"

"Mom, what are you talking about? Of course, I will find a job, but please do not even mention something else. I know exactly what you are trying to say. Being a young widow will not be easy, but my children's love will help me overcome all difficulties. I'm grateful for your help. I couldn't do this without you. But do not push; do not mention this again, please? I will never marry again. I hope you will never say this again. I love you, Mom."

Nora's mother looked down with tears in her eyes, hugged her daughter, and left her seat.

Bob and Ana were playing close to Nora. They came and hugged her then kissed her cheeks. It was like they knew what their grandmother talked to their mother about. When they were playing, the mailman brought an official letter and Nora had to sign for it. She signed it and went back to the bench to open and read it. She was terrified to open it. Who knows what "they" wanted from her now?

She asked her nephew Peter to read the letter to her.

He stared at his aunt wondering why she asked him to read the letter, but he did it. He opened the letter and started reading, "Mrs. Nora Salomea, according to our records, you are the recipient of your husband's life insurance, purchased November 1951. Soon you will receive a check in the mail. Sincerely yours."

If a pin had dropped, the entire house could have heard it. As Peter started reading the letter, Maria and their mother came closer to Nora, to listen while Peter read what the letter was all about. The silence after he finished was so deep, even the children seemed to realize something important had happened.

"Now I understand! Now I understand!" Nora screamed so loud that the kids got scared. She jumped up abruptly. "Now I see. How was it possible to not see his entire masterpiece, the planning to take his own life, so his family would have money to survive! It wasn't an accident; it was a suicide! No, wasn't just money, no. He couldn't live humiliated. He couldn't adapt to the new regime like so many others did. The party was his goodbye. It was his way of saying goodbye! It was his decision."

She grabbed the letter from her nephew's hands and she put it on her chest, crying. "I don't need your money; you are a coward, and your children needed you, not your money! I needed you, not your money. You left me alone with two children in a cruel world because you couldn't make it. Where was your love for us; how could you do this to us? All our friends and everybody in our family are trying hard to adapt to the new rules, but you couldn't. Coward, coward. It is hard; it will be hard, but they are alive, and now you are dead! How could you think that money could replace love! Why didn't you open your heart and talk to me? How was this possible when you knew very well how much I loved you? With shop or no shop, with money or no money, you were the love of my life. I loved you so much."

Nora kissed her children, and she asked her mother to watch them for a few hours. She needed to be alone, to cry her heart out.

Maria was afraid for her sister, afraid she might do something stupid, being so desperate. She let her go inside, and after a few minutes, Maria followed Nora into her room and stayed with her the whole time Nora wanted to be there.

Seeing her sister coming in her room, Nora was grateful. She wasn't angry or upset. She knew she would do the same thing for Maria.

When Nora woke up later, the words from the letter were

dancing in front of her eyes. Her mind was busy, thinking loud, *Who are you to judge Titus, God? Are you God? Who gave you the right to judge him? Why would he have to be like everybody else? Why would he have to think and behave like you or your friends? He was unique in his way; he was weaker than most people you know. It was his way of living on this earth; it was his own way of leaving this earth! You cannot judge him; we all are created differently, and God choose Titus's life and he gave him everything he needed. It was Titus's choice.*

Nora shook her head and prayed, talking to God like never before.

She stood up, straightened her body, and closed the door, She went to be with her kids and her family. She knew she left another world behind that door, and she knew God would bring another world for her and her children.

* * * *

One year after Titus passed, Nora had taken a job as an accountant's assistant at a pharmaceutical company, and her life was her children.

Bob and Ana were good students, and they played together with their neighbors. But both of them missed their father's love and the time they used to play. It was different from playing with their friends.

One day, Nora decided to take her children to visit their grandfather who had moved back to his home in the village. He had hoped, after doing so, there would be less painful memories. Nora insisted he could live with them, but he wanted to go back to his home. When Nora shared her intention with her kids, the joy was out of this world. They jumped up and down, happy to see their grandfather. It was a few hours trip by train.

Nora got chills just thinking about being on a train! Painful memories came to her mind. But she told herself that life goes on, and she needed to take the kids to see their grandfather.

She arrived at Simon's home and realized how sad everything

was. She felt good for bringing the kids there, seeing how the visit lifted their grandfather's spirits. They had a good time and Nora promised to visit again, when time and money would let her do it.

After a few months, she received a phone call. Because her father-in-law moved back to his country home, he needed to take care of some legal issues: his will, the house, and a lot more. Titus had been the only child, so now Nora was the only one to help. The children were in school so she had to go alone. She told her family what she needed to do, and everybody offered to help with the kids and the house. Nora's mother was getting older, but she was still doing things around the house and seemed to be ok. And, Maria was the stone of the family; she was the one everybody looked to, to ask for help. Nora was so blessed to have them.

She said goodbye and asked her children to be good and to listen to whatever their aunt and grandmother told them to do. She knew that Peter would be in charge when it came to their homework. She knew he would do a better job than she would and was so grateful for it.

Nora arrived at the station and waited for her train. When she got to her seat, she realized how crowded the cabin was. All men and no room enough between seats. It looked disgusting. She looked around and almost wanted to stand at the window but remembered it was a few hours' trip, so she took her seat. It seemed this day when Nora took the train, it was God's day off!

Nora was wearing black from head to toe, not even a trace of makeup, no jewelry, not one drop of femininity was transpiring from her body. Elegant, distinctive, pale, and full of dignity, she was the perfect picture of a widow or of somebody who had a recent death in her life.

Nora's seat was next to a man, and she tried to see if there were other seats, but all were taken. So she had no choice but to sit next to him. Thank God, she had only one side to worry about. The other side was next to the door. She was holding her arms close to her body, not wanting to touch that man, and she kept looking down. After a while, she started reading the book she brought with her, trying to concentrate on what she was reading. It was impossible to not see how uncomfortable she was.

The cabin was so crowded that Nora had no air to breathe, or it might have been because she felt so uneasy. She promised to herself to not do this again, noting how different it was from when she had the kids with her.

Finally, she arrived at her destination. After visiting with her father-in-law, her heart was even heavier. Titus's father was living like a dead man. Losing his only child, his only son, he lost everything. He was lost. Nora asked him again to come and live with her and the grandchildren, but he refused.

He knew his days were gone, his end was getting closer, and he didn't want to be a burden on her. She had enough. "Nora, I appreciate you asking me to come and live with you and the kids, but it is too late for me. I want to be buried next to my wife, Titus's mother. I love you and my grandchildren very much."

Nora took care of all the documents her father-in-law needed, making his life easier. She said a very sad goodbye to the man that was her husband's father. She was still married in her mind, and she thought she always would be.

Going towards the train station, she noticed something weird, as if a shadow was following her. Nora turned her head and recognized the man that had been sitting next to her in the train cabin. She considered that the man got off at the same stop and followed her to her in-law's house, waiting for her all that time. How did he know that she would be back? How did he know that she didn't live there?

Her hands started shaking; she felt furious and scared at the same time. What if he was a criminal? Where had he stayed when she was at her father-in-law's home? Why did he follow her? Did he watch every step she made? She thought about stopping at the police station, but what reasons did she have? She would be ok, once she got on the train and forgot about this incident. Hopefully, he lived here and would stay here.

Without turning her head or looking around, she got in the train, found her seat, and thanked God that the cabin was not crowded like when she first came. She grabbed her book and started reading, so the time would go faster. She forgot about that man, but when she got off the train, she could still feel that shadow behind her.

Nora got home and her children were all over her, happy to see their mom back. They asked about their grandfather and asked to visit him during summer vacation. She promised to take them to stay with their grandfather for a full month. This made them very happy.

As soon as she took care of her kids then talked to Maria and her mom, telling them about her father-in- law, her sadness was making her depressed and unhappy.

Titus and their love was everywhere. *My God, I still love him so much. He was my life, my mind, my heart, everything. I love him so much. Every second he is with me, I feel him around me.*

* * * *

Nora went to work every day and in the afternoon, she spent time with her kids and her family.

One day, she was heading to the tram station early in the morning and was in a hurry to not be late at work. She almost stopped when she noticed the *shadow* who followed her the last time she was on the train. Coming back from work, the man was there waiting. She tried to not look at him, to not make eye contact, but she was scared.

A few days went by and Nora didn't say one word about it to anybody, not even to Maria. She didn't want to bother her family with something she considered stupid. A few days in a row, the man always seemed to be where she was. Nora intended to go to the first police station she saw and report the situation, but she was concerned they would laugh at her story, so she never went.

"The policeman will say that he never hurt me, he never touched me, and who knows what else. And he would be right, but it makes me feel so uncomfortable," Nora kept telling herself.

The man knew Nora's schedule, her children's names, and her family members' names. He was there all the time, like he didn't have anything else to do.

* * * *

One day, he approached Maria. He introduced himself as being a construction engineer, being single, and in love with her sister Nora.

First, Maria didn't want to talk to this man; it was very impolite to stop a woman and introduce yourself. Her husband could kill him for what he did. Thank God, John didn't see the scene. She tried to keep going, but there was something about this man. He was very presentable, elegant, and clean.

She said, "Sir, I don't know you. Please leave and let my sister alone. She is mourning her husband. Respect her pain, please."

"Ma'am, I promise I will respect this. I will be back in a couple of months."

He said goodbye and kept his promise.

Nora had forgotten about him completely until one day when she saw him again, in the same place, waiting for her to go to the tram station. She was determined to tell Maria about what was going on. She took care of her kids, checked their homework, prepared all they would need for the next day, and put them to bed before going to Maria's home.

Maria and John were ready to go to bed when they heard somebody knocking at the door.

John went to check and saw Nora there. He opened the door and invited his sister-in-law to come inside.

She did, and Maria offered her a cup of tea. It was a chilly evening.

"What has happened? Is everybody ok?" Maria asked.

"Yes, thank God. I am so sorry to bother you, but I have to talk to you, both of you."

"Sit down and let's talk," John offered.

"I will not keep you long. You are so tired." Nora looked as worried as she sounded.

"We're not tired when it comes to our family," Maria insisted.

Nora's heart was full of love and gratitude for being blessed with such a family. Her brother-in-law was treating her like a real sister. John pulled a chair for Nora to sit down.

"There's a man," Nora started.

"A man?" Maria and John both asked.

"Yes, there's a man watching me all the time, every day. Not from a window, but in person, keeping the distance. I'm scared for my children's lives and for all of us. He could be a criminal."

"Nora, criminals don't act like this," John said. "They don't want you to see them. It seems like this man wants you to see him. But keep talking."

"When I went to visit Titus's father, my seat was next to this man's seat. He followed me to my father-in-law's house, and when I left the place to come back home, he was in the same train with me. He followed me all the way home, and since then, I see him all the time. I'm very scared. Please, help me. Titus, where are you? Why did you leave me?" Nora began to cry. Her body was shaking and she cried heavily.

John and Maria let her cry; she needed that relief. They looked at each other wondering how serious the problem was.

Maria wrapped her arms around Nora's shoulders and said, "Nora, let me take you home; get a good night's sleep. then tomorrow, we will see what has to be done about this situation."

John and Maria took Nora back home, and when they returned to their own home, they started talking instead of going to bed.

"John, what do you think? I'm speechless. Do you think she can be in danger?" At that moment, Maria was scared to tell her husband that she'd already talked to that man, so she pretended like it never happened.

"Take it easy! I will be in charge. Tomorrow, I will see what is going on. I promised Titus I would take care of his family like it is my own, and he promised me the same. Now go to bed and sleep. You work so hard."

Maria followed her husband's advice and went to bed; she was exhausted.

* * * *

John wasn't able to put it out of his mind, though. He was worried that it could be a serious situation and maybe he should call the police.

The next morning, he could see what Nora was talking about.

It was nearly time for Nora to leave the house and go to work. A tall, handsome man was walking up and down the street, watching their gate, where Nora should show up in a couple of minutes.

John kept watching through the window. He couldn't believe he hadn't noticed this man earlier, even though the school made the street they lived on busy. "I'm going to talk to that man, to see what is going on."

"No, please, don't go. Who knows what could happen?" Maria told her husband.

"I will be ok. Look how many parents are bringing their children to school. I have to talk to this man." Without waiting for Maria's permission, John left the house, crossed the street, and approached the man.

"Hi, what are you doing here, watching our yard? Are you waiting for somebody?"

"Yes, sir; by the way, my name is Nick. What is yours?"

"It isn't your business. You have to leave right now, or I will call the police. There are children going to school, and it isn't your place to stand here."

"Sir, I will leave soon because I have to go to work, but I will be back this afternoon. I don't mean any harm to anybody."

John had to admit the man was right, but still he wanted him out of his sight.

"Sir, I love a woman that lives in the same yard with you. She has two children and I think she lost her husband. Actually, she is leaving the house right now." John turned his head and he saw Nora coming out of her house.

She was wearing black, head to toe, distinctive and simple. She looked for a second at John and the man. She continued walking without looking surprised. She didn't say one word. She didn't even greet her brother-in-law, but she did walk faster than normal.

"Nick, or whatever your name is, leave right now and don't ever come back here. I will call the police."

"I'll leave right now, but you don't need the police. I am a respectable man. I have a good job, and the only thing I ask for, is to meet this lady and talk to her." Nick said goodbye and left.

* * * *

John went inside the house where Maria was hidden behind the curtains. She watched everything but she couldn't wait to see what John was going to say. When John opened the door, she started asking questions, "Who is this man? What does he want? Why did you talk to him so long?"

"He wants Nora. His answers were prompt and simple. This is what he wants."

"Nora? What does he have to do with my sister?"

"Don't you remember what your sister told us last night when she came over?"

"Oh, now I see! I hope you told him to not ever come back."

"How did you know? That is exactly what I said. But his answer was polite and firm. He told me again that he wants to meet Nora and talk to her."

"Did you tell him she just lost her husband?"

"No, I didn't. I wasn't going to have a conversation with him, but I did say that if he keeps coming back and watching our yard, I will call the police."

"Good, perfect. Let's see if he comes back." Maria felt like a heavy stone was lifted from her shoulders, realizing the man didn't say one word about their meeting. In truth, she'd almost forgotten about the incident, being busy with her life.

Later that afternoon, the streets were less busy. The kids had already left school and less people were in the street. Only the occasional tram or trolleybus ran up or down the street to bring people home from work.

Suddenly, the man showed up. He was wearing an elegant suit, and as soon as he reached his point of observation, he lifted his hat to greet the "invisible" people that he knew were watching behind the curtains. He stood there for a few minutes, lifted his hat again, and left.

Maria and John had no idea how to deal with such a situation. Maria wasn't sure if Nora should know about the conversation between John and Nick. Especially, now that they had his name.

Both of them decided that it wasn't the right moment to talk to Nora about how much this man wanted to meet her. She was still so much in love with Titus, and it seemed she would always be.

* * * *

Nora was getting better, though at least, she'd started smiling again. The children were the ones making her happy. With four kids around her, taking care of homework, sports and being playful with them, there wasn't too much time left to think about your own problems; and for Nora, this was a blessing. She remembered the proverb: "busy minds, happy minds."

Ana and Bob were mentioning their father's name often, especially when they were playing. Titus spoiled his kids a lot and let his wife be the educator—the same situation from Nora's family. Her mother had been the tough one and her father had spoiled the children. Bob had his father's image in his young mind. You could see on his face how much he missed his father. Nora tried hard to recreate Titus's attitude when playing with her children, but she wasn't successful. She noticed how at certain times of the day, like when Titus used to come home, Bob and Ana would look towards the gate, waiting for their father to come home.

It was a heart-breaking image, to see her children missing their father. Thank God for Maria and their big family. She couldn't imagine how her life would be without them.

* * * *

Even though Nick kept coming by in recent months, John never got the police involved, knowing the man was innocent, that he wasn't doing anything wrong. "Maria, we need to tell Nora about what this man wants and let her decide."

"Are you crazy? She is a widow."

"I know it, but she is a young widow, with two children to take care of. We protect them, love them, but they need a father. What about if we have to move to another city? What if I get another job somewhere else?"

"What? Are we moving?"

"No, Maria, you didn't listen to me! I said, *if.* Who is going to look after these kids? They're growing so fast. Look at our Peter; he's almost a man now."

"Let's hope that man has good intentions for my sister and my nephew and my niece. I love them like I love my own kids."

"So, what do you suggest?"

"You're right; it is the time to talk to her. I am afraid it will be the first time she will hate me. She's still in love with her husband, but you are so right; she has to think further. She will need somebody to raise those kids, to love them and to support her own family, even if we will also be taking care of them. She needs somebody. She is so young."

That evening, after the children went to bed and everything was put back in order for the next day, Maria and John went to Nora's home.

They had a long conversation about a subject that was unexpected and unwelcome for Nora. She couldn't believe that her own sister would talk about such a thing...the man who was watching her like an eagle. "What? You want me to talk to that man? Why? I don't want to talk to anybody. I don't need to talk to him. I hate that man. And I will call the police. This subject is over, I promise."

They hadn't expected such a strong reaction from Nora. Maria and John left and they didn't exchange one word.

Getting home, a few feet away from Nora's home, they said their prayers and went to bed, concerned about Nora's future.

* * * *

Ultimately, Nora never called the police. She got so used to seeing the man standing there, in front of their yard, like a light pole or a tree.

Every time she left home, the man was lifting his hat, greeting her with respect. She did notice how handsome he was, but she didn't like him or the way he behaved.

One day, John stopped and asked the man, "Are you still here?"

"Yes, sir, I will be here till I get a chance to talk to the beautiful lady that lives across the street."

"She's my wife!" John tried to see what the man knew.

"No, sir, your wife is taller and you have two boys. My lady is shorter, and she has a boy and a girl."

"How come you know all of these things? Do you spy on us?"

"No, but when I'm waiting to see my lady, I can see other things too. Please, let me talk to her and I promise I won't do anything wrong. I respect this lady, and I'm in love with her even though we have never talked."

"Nick—can you believe I remembered your name? Do you have a few minutes to talk?"

"Yes, sir, I manage a big construction company and I have people that can take care of things when I'm not there."

"Ok. Let's talk."

They started walking up the street. It was a beautiful street, windy and lined with many homes. It had been really beautiful before the war and the street's name, Trinity, saved many of its houses from being destroyed by bombs. At least, the people living there thought that way. They'd been blessed that most of the beautiful houses were still standing. Jewish and Christian people were living together in harmony, being a real example for most of the other neighborhoods.

John was asking a myriad of questions, without giving Nick one chance to ask even one question. At the end of their walk, John was satisfied with all the answers he received from Nick. "I have to leave now, and I cannot promise anything."

"I do appreciate you giving me the opportunity to talk to you. Thank you for taking the time. I will be here like a sentinel at the queen's palace," Nick said, smiling.

John smiled too.

Nick's heart was beating about a hundred miles per hour. He was so happy that he finally got a chance to "talk" in a civilized manner with somebody from her family. His day was like no other day, smiling and agreeing with everybody. People noticed something different in his behavior. He couldn't wait for the work day to be over so he could go back to his "love."

* * * *

"Maria, Nora, Mom, come here, please, we need to talk."

"What's so urgent?" Maria asked him. "You haven't even hugged your kids!"

"Don't worry. I will do it later on."

"Go ahead," his mother-in-law. Linda urged. John called her 'Mom' because she was a real mom, a good mother for all of them, especially for her grandchildren.

"Nora, this meeting is for you. I know it is not my job to get involved in your business, but do you remember what I said when Titus passed away? I promised to take care of you and your children. Before I start talking, I just want to reassure everybody how much I love each of you."

"Ok, what is this all about?" Nora felt she knew the subject already and was ready to leave the room.

"Nora, do you remember that man that I told you about? His name is Nick, and I had a long conversation with him today."

"I don't care. I don't want to hear one word about him or why he's here all the time. He is a predator."

"He already knows you're a widow and that you have two children."

"So, if he knows all these things, why does he still stand out there all the time? He's disturbed. Nobody normal would do what he does. I don't care about him or anybody else. I don't need a man in my life. I still love my husband, even if he was a coward."

"We know how much you still love Titus," John replied. "But you're so young and your kids need a father in their lives. Maybe it is hard to see this now, but later on in life, you will realize what I mean. I only try to show you how hard it will be to raise your beautiful children without a father. Everybody needs a human being in their lives to share the good and the bad; we all need a shoulder to cry on."

"I have a family…you are my family. I love you all one by one. Your children are my children, and I know how much you love my children. Am I wrong?"

"John is right," Linda said. "You are right too, but give him a chance to explain."

The silence shut them all down. Nobody ever expected the frail woman, the tiny woman who was the foundation of her family, to even know about this subject. They assumed she had no idea about the man watching Nora. But she knew exactly what was going on, daily. She knew more about the man than John, because she could read people and their intentions.

Nora knew the shock and surprise she felt was pointless when she looked at her mother and figured out her mom had always been watching, every time she left for work. She'd been there all the time, to be sure her daughter was safe. Nora felt more amazed than ever. She remembered the proverb of *who doesn't have old people, should buy them!* How true this was.

Nora listened to her mom and let John explain the whole situation with that weird man. "Ok, John, I'm ready to listen to you."

Nora listened to John's speech about "the statue" without interrupting.

There were no comments. Nobody dared to say something. Everybody went back to whatever they'd been doing before the meeting.

The seed had been planted.

CHAPTER SEVEN

Nora hugged everybody, wishing them good night, and she started getting ready for the night. She was like a robot, doing things automatically. In the back of her mind, she knew she had to do something for her children's future and for herself. She knew how hard it was, and would be to raise her children as a single parent. These times weren't like it used to be before the war.

The country needed more time to recover, to rebuild. Her city was still in bad shape. People had to work hard to make a living and most of them found work on the construction sites, where the government was building tall, ugly apartments, where they could put people to live while confiscating their homes. She was lucky to have even found a good job as an accountant's assistant at a pharmaceutical company and get a salary to raise her children. She wanted her kids to grow healthy and strong. Images of them playing together in the years ahead blossomed in her mind.

"Why should I change their lives? Who gives me this right? I am their mom, not God. Why should I change what we have? Why should I bring a stranger in our family? Who needs a man? Not me, that's for sure!" But somewhere, far away in her mind a thought was coming to the surface. *I am young. I need a man. No, I don't! I hate these thoughts. I have my children. Who knows how my kids will be treated by another man?*

What about when your children get older and leave the house, having their own families with kids, what are you going to do alone?

"Oh, I will be old by then," Nora now spoke aloud. "What about till then? " She shook her head. "Absolutely not! I don't need another man in my life or my children's lives. We are happy the way we are." She felt new determination to tell this man to stop coming, that she wasn't interested in talking to or seeing him. Enough was enough.

Tomorrow would be the last day she ever saw him.

* * * *

After her children left for school, Nora grabbed her purse and left to go to work. The man was there, like always, holding a huge bouquet of flowers. Nora went directly to him, looked him in his eyes, then with a mean look and an iced voice, she said, "Sir, please, do not ever come back here. I don't want to see you anymore. I do not need you or anyone else in my life. I have my children and my family. Respect my wishes and forget about this place."

"Yes, ma'am, I will respect you and your family. Please accept these flowers and give me permission to come once in a while? If only to see you from the distance. I promise to not bother you anymore. I want you to know that I love you. I'll still come, but I will hide from your sight."

Nora couldn't believe what she just heard. How could you love somebody you don't even know? But she remembered the same thing had happened with Titus. He was in love with her from the second he looked at her. She accepted the flowers, thinking they had no fault, and said, "As long as I don't see you here, you can do whatever you want." She turned around, holding the flowers, and went back inside the house to put them in a vase.

The family watched from behind their curtains. They saw the flowers and Nora accepting them, and everybody was surprised but hoping that maybe the day would come.

The flowers reminded Nora of the "good times" when Titus would come home with his arms full of flowers in carriages pulled by horses. What times they had. Her love for Titus was stronger than ever. Her eyes were full of tears.

* * * *

Nora was taking care of things, even being promoted at work. Her boss was very happy with her skills. Nora's brain was fast and quick. Ana and Bob were growing like weeds. She couldn't stop thinking of what John had told her about her future.

She knew he was right. "Look how fast those kids have grown. They are so big. Soon they will be taller than me! I think Bob is already taller than me," she told herself.

Nora's heart was telling her to accept this man, at least get to know him. Even if he was tall and handsome, Nora knew she wasn't attracted to him. She remembered how she felt when she saw Titus for the first time. The earth shook! And she had a completely opposite feeling looking at this man. She wanted to run away from him—far, far, away.

Of course, it was flattering to see how much admiration he had for her. It was impressive to see him every day, sometimes twice a day, standing there like a statue, waiting to see her. All her neighbors had noticed the man and the fact he was all eyes for Nora.

Maria talked a few times with her sister about being willing to talk to the man, to see if she would like him. "Nora, this man loves you. Just talk to him; maybe become friends? He seems to be so lonely."

"Why don't you talk to him if you feel so sorry for him?"

Maria frowned at her sister's tone. "Nora, get real. You will need somebody, someday."

"Maybe I will need somebody in my life. I know I'm young, but I still love Titus. I can't even look at that man."

The man had no idea how many people talked to Nora on his behalf. But life continued to go on and day by day, the things that needed done... got done. Bob and Ana were lucky to have their cousins, playing together. They were four amazing children, loving each other like brothers and sisters. It was a blessing for everybody to see them so close and happy.

The day came when Nora said to Maria, "Ok, I am feeling so down. Thank God for all of you. I think I'll listen to you and John. Go and talk to that man. He does look clean, and he is handsome. His skin is so much lighter than mine."

Maria was so excited to hear what her sister just said. She ran inside to tell John.

Her mother, of course, already knew it…it was called a mother's intuition.

Nora crossed the street, knowing the man would show up. Shortly after, the man who had been waiting for this moment for a few months appeared in front of her.

"Hi, my name is Nora," she said. "I didn't tell you my name when we talked last time."

He lifted his hat, took Nora's hand and kissed it.

This didn't surprise Nora, because it was a common and polite gesture to kiss a woman's hand when a man greeted a woman.

"My name is Nick, and I'm very happy to talk to you, to meet you."

"I know you know that I have two children and I'm a widow."

"I know and I even know their names."

"How do you know their names?"

"I have heard their names when you or other relatives call them to come inside the house for dinner. I knew your name, too. I know everybody's name," he said, smiling.

"Oh, I see," Nora said.

They went for a walk that didn't last long, but long enough to agree to see each other again, for another walk.

* * * *

When Nora got home, Maria couldn't stop her curiosity. "So, what do you think about him? Was he polite?"

"Yes, very. We went for a walk and talked. He is a construction engineer and he is in charge of a large project for apartment buildings. I told him where I work and what I do there, a little bit about each of you, and of course, about all the kids and our parents. He already knew everybody's name. But this is enough for today. We'll see how things go." Nora put her arms around her sister's shoulders and looking in her eyes, she said, "I don't like this man. He cannot compare with Titus. Nobody can ever compare with him.

I still hate him for leaving me alone with two children in such difficult times. Maria, Titus loved us very much, but he was a weak man; he couldn't handle the new changes like most of us. I think I'm trying to give him an excuse. I love my husband."

"I understand Nora and you should do what will be best for you and your kids. Remember, the night is a good adviser. Get some rest, and I will see you tomorrow morning before going to work. I like having my coffee with you. Good night," she said, closing the door behind her.

When John came home from work, Maria greeted him by telling him all about the news that her sister finally talked to the man!

John couldn't believe it, but he seemed happy to hear it.

"John, Nora doesn't like the man; she was very clear about it."

"Don't worry. He's smart and good looking. It won't take long to see them together. He already told me that he was never married and he has no children. Do you think he is younger than Nora?"

"Even if he is, it doesn't make any difference. Nora is such a beautiful young woman. I know she's my sister, but we always agreed how beautiful she is."

"Absolutely, two gorgeous sisters," John said, pulling his wife closer to him. "I am so lucky."

Maria smiled and kissed her husband with love and passion.

* * * *

The next day, Nick was in the same place, waiting for Nora to give him a sign that they could talk. Nora accepted Nick's every offer to go for longer walks, and she became more comfortable in his presence. One afternoon, they went to see a movie. Nora was afraid that Nick would try to get closer to her, but he kept a decent distance and didn't touch her at all. She felt impressed with his behavior, so she accepted another invitation from him.

Marrying Nora was the only thing Nick wanted. He knew she had two children, and he was ready to give them his name, to become their father.

Nora was taken by surprise one afternoon when Nick proposed.

She couldn't answer. She ran home, crying. She stopped at Maria's home and thanked God that she was there. Nora needed her. "How can I, how can I?" Nora kept saying.

"Can, what? Nora, what's going on; why are you crying? Talk to me." Maria asked all these questions, thinking Nick did something wrong.

"Maria, he asked me to marry him," Nora said through tears.

"Oh, thank God, it isn't something bad."

"What else could it be?" Nora asked, looking at her sister.

"I thought he had hurt you."

"Oh, no, he didn't! He is so polite."

"What did you answer?"

"Answer? I didn't answer. I ran home!"

"Well, then, you should go home, relax, then ask yourself what you want for you and for your children. Tomorrow, your mind and heart will be clearer and you can be sure what you have to do. Nobody has the answer but you alone. Good night. Love you, sister, very much."

Nora left, but she knew the answer. "Why? Why?" she asked herself. "I need to marry him for my children, even if I'm not attracted to him. My kids need a father. I know that this might be the wrong reason, but…"

The next time they met, Nick asked the question again.

Nora looked at him and said, "I want you to meet my family, my parents, my sister and her family and above all, my children."

They went inside the house where Nora's kids were playing. Homework was done and they enjoyed running around the living room, making lots of noise, a very happy noise.

When the door opened and Nora and Nick entered the room, the children stopped and looked at each other, wondering who this person was.

Their mother approached Bob and said, "Bob, this is Mr. Nick and he is a good friend of mine."

Bob shook Nick's hand like he was taught to do, but his face had no smile on it.

Ana came closer after she heard what her mom said to Bob.

Nora hugged her and said, "Ana, this is Mr. Nick, a good friend of mine."

Ana went behind her mother's legs, hiding.

Nora then introduced Nick to her parents. They had known of him for a long time, but not officially.

Nick brought flowers, wine, and chocolate. He handed the chocolate box to Bob, but he refused to take it.

Nora, noticing Bob's gesture, said to Nick, "My children are so young; they will need time to get to know you."

Nick didn't stay long; he said good night and left.

Bob looked at his mother and asked, "Why did he come in our home?"

"Bob, Mr. Nick is a good man and he wants to spend more time with you and your sister, so you can become friends."

"Ok, I hope we can play like two men."

"Ana, why did you hide? Mr. Nick wants to get to know you."

"Mom, he is a stranger. How can I play with a stranger?"

"Ana, a stranger is a person in the street that you don't know, but if a person is invited into your home, he is a guest. Mr. Nick was my guest."

Ana looked at Bob and both of them agreed to be nice to him the next time he visited.

* * * *

Nora and Nick got married on a rainy day. No loud music, not too many people. It was a quiet wedding. Nick's heart was very happy.

Nora's heart was somewhere else, but she was content thinking of her children's future.

Soon, Bob and Ana realized that Mr. Nick would be their father from now on. Ana was way too young to realize the difference between the father she knew and loved and this "new father," but Bob had already noticed that the new father spent a lot more time with his mom than talking to or playing with them. Nora compensated for that time though, spending all the time she had with her kids. They were the best thing in her life and all that she had eyes for.

Nora's parents had a large property and as they had once worried, they'd been forced to accept a tenant in one of the rooms, a police officer. Nobody wanted the tenant, but he was sent there by the new regime, so he was accepted in silence. The rent he was paying was close to nothing. If Nora's parents refused the new tenant, they could be considered enemies of the Communist Party.

So, they kept their mouths shut and signed the papers.

That had only been the beginning; an official letter came. And Nora's parents started crying after they opened the letter and read it. They almost had heart attacks.

"Mom, what's wrong? Tell me, please!" Nora was upset by their behavior. "Mom, give me the letter you hold in your hand. Father, please, sit down; I am scared of the way your faces look." She grabbed the letter to start reading it. Nora's face became paler and paler. The letter informed her parents, the owners of the property, that soon they would receive a new place to live, in an apartment building, because the state needed their property. It was the cruelest letter they had ever received. They would be sent to a place where they have to pay rent, not own it, and receive a minor financial compensation.

After reading the letter, Nora told them not to worry, that the letter was a scam, a joke, a very bad joke. She asked her parents to calm down and not to take it seriously.

* * * *

Later, during the day, Maria was stopped in the street by one of her neighbors. She was glad to see her friend and neighbor, to chat a little.

Her friend had tears in her eyes and her face looked terrified.

"What's happened to you? Why are you crying? What's wrong? Do you need help?" Maria asked.

"No," her friend answered. "Did you receive the letter?"

"What letter?"

"Look and read it." The neighbor gave Maria the letter and she could not stop crying.

When Maria finished reading, she excused herself and ran to her home. As soon as opened the door, she went directly to her parents. "Did you receive the letter?" Maria asked her mom.

"Yes, we did, but Nora told us to take it easy—maybe it is a scam or a joke."

"Mom, it is not a scam and it's not a joke. This is the new way; this is how the Communist Party confiscates properties, so they can build whatever they want without paying much for it."

"So, you think this is real?"

"Yes, other neighbors got the same thing."

"Tomorrow, we'll go to City Hall and see what all this is about. They cannot do this to people. This cannot be true."

Maria let her mom think that the letter wasn't so serious, so as not hurt them more. She told Nora, Nick, and John to follow her into another room. The children were quiet in their rooms, reading.

They talked about the letter and the new situation.

"What about our children? They would have to change schools," Nora said without addressing her question to anybody in particular. "How can we live in a tiny apartment with two kids?" She knew from Nick how small those apartments were and how far away they were from their place. "Maria, what are we going to do? This will kill our parents."

Maria was shocked and couldn't talk.

Nick and John were sitting around the table, speechless.

Nick finally said, "The apartments we build are located outside the capital, in the suburbs. They're very small. They make us work hard, even overtime, so they can get rid of the central houses and build elegant villas for their own people, important members of the new regime. If some of the houses' owners refuse to cooperate, they can be put in prison or— well, this is a very serious matter, and it will change lives forever. It will be hard, especially for your parents."

Everybody knew he was right. They had been seeing all of these changes around them, but, like always, people ultimately believed these kinds of tragedies wouldn't touch them, only somebody else, until it did.

That time came, having to accept an apartment for each family. They had to move and leave everything behind. Nora knew this move would destroy her parents. To confiscate their home and make them pay rent was too much to handle at their age.

In a bittersweet moment, Maria and Nora's mother passed away before she had to see this disaster. It was a tragedy. They lost the pillar of their family; they lost the grandmother of their kids! Those kids had been hurt again. Their grandmother, the one they went to for comfort and everything else they needed when their parents weren't there, especially Bob and Ana. It was one tragedy after another. God had to give them a break, but the break was far away—very far away.

Nora's heart was broken. She lost her mother, her children lost their favorite person on Earth, and after losing their father—and, on top of everything, the kids and Nick didn't get along. Her marriage wasn't what she hoped for. Nick was a very cold man: an iceberg, she called him in her mind. Nick liked the children and he tried hard to be a good father, but something was always missing…love! He didn't have kids and he had no idea how to attract a child to make him or her love him. All his attention was for Nora and he loved her. But children were like small animals; they could feel if you loved them or not. Nick knew that if he wanted to win Nora's love, he had to win her children first. Working long hours, coming home late, most of the time, the kids were already sleeping, so they grew apart from him.

"God, I lost my love, my husband, and now my mom; and my marriage is falling apart. God, do something, please. On top of everything, I am losing my home now."

Maria and John had a really tough time accommodating themselves to the new changes. Maria was very close to her mom, learning everything she knew from her. They had helped and relied on each other so much, she grew up being more like her mom's sister. She had to go and spend some time with her sister, so they could cry on each other's shoulders.

She went to Nora's home and, without saying one word, they hugged each other, crying until they felt lighter.

Nobody, not even their children, interrupted their mourning.

* * * *

They signed the lease agreements and started packing with tears in their eyes.

This was the house where they'd been born, their kids had been born there too. All the happy and sad events had taken place in that house.

The tenant knew about this change a long time in advance, and he asked his boss to make him a tenant in their house, so he would get an apartment when the house was confiscated. The government planned this move a long time ago.

Now Nora and Maria could see all the dirt, at least from their level.

Maria got an apartment in a much better building than Nora. Maria's apartment building had some grass outside and it seemed to be a quiet neighborhood. Nora's apartment was on the last floor and extremely small. She went to City Hall to complain about the size and the location of the new apartment, but the answer she received made her realize how strong this regime was. She knew she had to accept it or be in the street. She would find a way to survive in the apartment, looking only a little bit better than a prison.

She had to find a way; her children had to be happy.

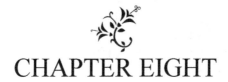

CHAPTER EIGHT

The family was separated now. Nora's and Maria's children changed schools.

Different schools, different teachers, different students, no friends. Nora and Maria could see their children weren't as happy as they used to be and this bothered them.

They were just starting to get used to the new situation when Nick came home and announced that they would have to move to another city, where his job would be. It was such a shock that Nora refused to believe this could happen to her and her children again. Ana and Bob would have to move again, change again, after only just getting used to the new teachers, the new students.

Nora knew she had to follow her husband and take her children with her because her mother was gone. If she were still alive, she would let the children stay with their grandmother, to take care of them. Bob could help with Ana's homework, being smart and an excellent student. But there was no solution, her mom was dead and nothing could change her fate.

Maria couldn't believe she would have no sister to talk to, to cry together, and to help each other.

Both of the sisters talked to God, using big words and asking for things that couldn't happen and they knew it. Things were getting harder and harder.

The lack of love grew deeper between Nick and the children. It didn't help when their family started moving from one city to another, with each move meaning a new school, new teachers, and new students. They had become like gypsies, moving from one place to another, destroying any sense of stability. Nora's children grew up without the deep roots they had before their mother married Nick.

Nora started thinking about going back to her hometown, finding a place to live and take care of her family on her own. She didn't love her husband, but she didn't care about love anymore; it was about seeing what was happening to Bob and Ana. Nora and Nick lived like roommates, but were still a married couple.

Maria missed her sister and her nephew and her niece. They were far apart and there was no easy way to communicate between them. Maria knew how miserable her sister was, unhappy and the worst was the situation with Bob and Ana. Maria's children had a better chance; they didn't have to move or leave the town. They were able to have steady friends and a much better life. Bob and Ana were never able to make friends, moving so often and so many times. But they had each other and Nora was so grateful to see them happy together.

It didn't take Nick long to begin insisting they have a child, but Nora didn't want to have another child. Times were hard and the situation between them wasn't the best. Nick didn't see their marriage the same way; he thought everything was going well. He didn't spend too much time at home, being all day long on the construction site.

After a few more months among strangers, they came back to Bucharest, grateful to be reunited with Maria and her family. The children were happy to be in their city, the city they loved. Things seemed to get better just for being back in their own environment.

* * * *

"Oh, no! Not now! God, please, don't let this happen to me. God, please, not now." Nora felt desperate—she was pregnant! This was so different from the way she felt the first time she found out she was pregnant. She remembered how happy she'd been with both pregnancies. No, this could not be happening to her. She didn't need another child; times were so hard to raise a child, to offer the baby all the things a baby needs, including love. "I don't love my husband. I cannot have his child. I have to do something; I have to ask Maria to help me." There was no way Nora could accept having another child.

* * * *

Maria finished her work day and went home, happy but tired. She loved helping women, making their lives easier. Everybody she met, everybody she worked with, loved her. There was something about her that made people happy to be around her. She was so grateful Nora and her family moved back to Bucharest, so she could have them closer. The cousins had missed each other and their time together. As soon as she got home, the phone rang.

"Maria, thank God you are home. I have to talk to you; it is urgent!"

Maria couldn't understand one word from what Nora was saying. "Nora, please, calm down. What's happened? Are you ok? What about the children? Nora, please talk to me."

"No, I cannot say it over the phone. You know how they listen to everything we talk about on the phone. May I come now?"

"What question is this? Did we ask each other such a thing when we had a problem, because it seems like we have a problem. I say 'we' because if you have a problem, I have a problem too. Hurry up; I'll wait for you with a nice dinner. Nora, have you served dinner to your family? We could spend more time together, if you have."

"Ok, you're right. I will do it. I'll be there in a heartbeat. See you soon."

* * * *

Nora arrived looking like she saw a ghost, pale and her eyes were swallowed by shadows. She looked desperate and lost.

Maria invited her inside and hugged her with love. She was so happy to have her sister in her apartment, like years before.

Maria got tears in her eyes remembering their beautiful house and how they lived there, all the children together and having their parents to help them. Now the situation was so different. Separated from each other, living in a much smaller place, but love is love. It didn't matter where you lived. How you felt about loving your family never changes. She realized her sister was in need of comfort, so she came back to reality. "Come and sit down, here, close to the heater. It is cold outside."

"Maria, I need your help, now!"

"What's happened? Is it Nick?"

"No, I am pregnant and you have to help me to do something. You know very well what I mean." Nora couldn't stop talking, feeling desperate, devastated.

"Did you just find out? Are you sure? Does Nick know about it? You know how much he wants a child of his own."

"No, nobody knows, you are the first and I hope the last one to find out. I don't want to have another child. I don't love Nick, and I do not want him to make differences between my children and his. He already doesn't pay attention to their education, and he's not a good father for my children. He is such a selfish man. It isn't right to bring another child in this world. The newborn will create problems in my family because Nick will have eyes only for his baby and completely neglect my children," Nora kept talking. "God, why did I marry that man? Why did my husband take his own life, leaving us so unhappy? I have to pay for my mistakes, I know it, but why the children? It isn't their fault. God help me to fix my mistakes, help my children. They are so innocent. Punish me, but help them."

"Nora, it isn't about what you think is right; it is what God wants for you and your family. Tell me why you feel this way about your husband? He seems to be a good, hard- working man that works hard to provide for all of you. Tell me what you don't like about him."

"Maria, I didn't come all the way here to talk about Nick. You have to help me. I will never have this baby. I refuse to have this baby. But I will answer your question, if I must. Nick knew from the beginning that I had two children, and he knew very well how much I adore my kids. He promised to be a good father for them, but he is distant. He's a cold father with no feelings. Bob and Ana feel the difference between Titus and Nick. My children feel the lack of love. The fact that he adopted them legally and they have his last name now, it didn't make any difference. It was just a paper."

"He will change now, when he becomes a real father," Maria stated. "He will have his own child and this will make him feel like a father and his behavior will change, believe me. You have to have this baby. Nora, this baby will be the glue needed in your family. Bob and Ana are such good children, so they will take care and love the baby and their feelings towards Nick will be different. You have to have this baby. You need this baby. God sent you this gift at the right moment. Now, you feel like everything is ruined, your life, your children's future. Nora, please listen to God, accept his gift, and go home with a heart full of hope and love. This baby is God's love caring for you and your family. It couldn't be a better time than now. God's timetable is a lot better than ours and we never know when it's coming. Open your heart and be thankful. I'm so happy for you and for your family. I couldn't come up with a better solution for your life. Remember, John and me, we will always be here for you. Go home now and tell them, or not? It is your decision. I know you will, though. I know what is in your heart. I love you, sister. Good night and see you soon."

Nora couldn't believe what just happened to her! How her sister's wisdom changed her completely. She remembered how she was feeling a few hours ago compared to how her attitude was now after talking to her sister. She thanked God all the way home for having such a sister. *Maria has become my mother and my sister in one person. What a blessing to have her in my life. I went to her apartment to ask her to get rid of my baby, and she convinced me to keep the baby!* Nora now felt blessed.

"Hi, Mom, where have you been?" Bob asked, hugging his mom.

"I had to go and see your aunt and talk to her. How was school? Did you do your homework? Did you help Ana to finish hers?"

"Of course, everything is done and Ana did all her homework by herself. She's a smart cookie," he said, smiling.

Ana came closer to them and hugged her mom like she hadn't

seen her for a very long time. "Mom, I miss you. Stay home. Don't go anywhere; stay with us."

"I miss you, too," Nora said and kissed both of them with so much love that she almost hurt them, but it was a good hurt, a mom's loving care, a mom's hurt.

Nick waited for the children to go to bed, anxious to talk to his wife. "Nora, are you ok? You don't look right. Did you cry? You look like you have cried. Nora, please, talk to me. I cannot stand to see you like this."

"Nick, I am pregnant."

"What?" he shouted, jumping from his chair. He hugged his wife's body and he was dancing all over the room. "You have no idea how much I wanted to hear this from your mouth. I always wanted a child from the moment I met you. I love you, Nora; I adore you."

"Nick, you have to treat all the children the same; do not make any differences among them. I'm afraid you will show more love to your child than to my children, and you will neglect them. Don't forget, children can feel it. Do not ever hurt them. They know who loves them and who doesn't. You have to spend more time with them, play together, and do things together."

"I promise I will do it. Nora, you have made me the happiest man in the world, thank you. I cannot wait to hold my baby in my arms. I adore you."

Nora started preparing Bob and Ana for receiving a new addition to their family.

Their reaction was pure happiness. When she saw this, her heart was full of hope and peace. She thanked her sister again, for what she did.

I know my kids. I know how I raised them and I know the education I gave them about family. My kids know that family is everything. They will love and protect the baby for the rest of their lives. I have to tell them that this baby will be their brother or sister. We will not use the words 'step,' or 'half,' the baby will be their brother or their sister. Actually, we have never had a similar situation in our family. I'm the only one who's ever remarried.

Nora thought about why she didn't feel like Nick was part of the family, why she didn't feel like he would be a good father. How she'd wished she never married him. It wasn't what she had dreamed for her children and for herself.

But life was going on, day by day. Nora kept very busy with her children's school, homework, sports, music, soccer, and all the things that come with having children of school age. One day, in the middle of the summer, a beautiful baby girl was born! She had huge dark eyes and lots of hair.

Maria helped Nora to deliver this sweet, adorable baby. "Nora, she is so beautiful; she looks just like you! Usually, girls look like their fathers, but this one looks like our children. I'm so happy for you. Let me take care of her, and then I will give her to you to hold her. I will take care of you, too, but she comes first." Maria was tired but happy. "Sophia will be our queen. I like her name."

"I like what you just said. I like this name too. Sophia will be her name. I can't wait to see my children's reaction. Chris was the youngest till now; Sophia is now the youngest. But I know Chris will love and spoil his new cousin. Maria, thank you for everything you did for me and for my children. Without you, Sophia wouldn't be here. Thank you from the bottom of my heart."

Bob and Ana were waiting outside to be allowed to see the baby and their mom. When the time came, both children were so anxious they tried to get through the door at the same time. Ana's eyes doubled in size! She couldn't take her eyes from the tiny doll—what she already decided to call her. Bob was the first one to hold Sophia. He was talking to her like he had known her forever.

Nora didn't even have a chance to hold her newborn baby girl. Bob and Ana were taking turns holding Sophia. Maria held the baby from underneath to be sure she was safe. Finally, Nora put the baby on her chest. The touch, the bonding, the feeling she had was out of this world, and reminded her of the times when she held Bob and Ana the same way.

Nora realized she'd been a lot happier back then, even if it was war and now was peace. Those were the kind of feelings she had in her heart when she had her older children and the love for Titus. She remembered her promise to herself that she would try the best she could to make them one happy family.

"Mom, thank you so much for giving us such a present," Ana said. "I always wanted to have a sister. Now I do. I'm so happy. I will help you raise her. I am old enough and I know how to do things. Aunt Maria told us her name—I love her name and I love my sister."

"I know you know, and I know you are going to help me with this baby. Isn't she precious? Look how beautiful she is. I think she looks like you, Ana!"

"I want her to look like you, but if she looks like me that's ok too."

* * * *

Nick went shopping for the new baby and to buy flowers for Nora. He stopped many times to share the news with his neighbors. His happiness was so obvious. "I'm a father. I have a daughter!" That's all what he could think about. What a beautiful girl and she is mine! I wonder why we cannot buy all that we need for the newborn before the baby was born. Who came up with this idea? So bad! I could spend all this time with Nora and Sophia instead of shopping!

Suddenly, he realized what his thoughts were just now… Nora and Sophia. Why he didn't think of Bob and Ana? "Why don't I feel the same love like I have for my new baby girl? They are such good children. They respect me; they've never talked back to me, and they call me dad! "Ok, Nick," he said to himself, "you have to change, to become a better father for these children, even if you love your own baby more." Nick promised himself he would try harder to be closer to Bob and Ana too. But, how many times had he already said this?

Nick bought everything on the list, went back home, and couldn't stop looking at his baby. Sophia was surrounded by love and care. She was the youngest in the family now and all the attention was for her. Ana and Bob were taking turns feeding her, changing her, taking her outside with the stroller. This child had the best life of all the kids in the family, and everybody loved her.

The only problem was that Nick's behavior was getting more and more obvious, treating his own child so much differently than the other two. Everybody thought it was because Sophia was so young, but even as she grew up, things were the same. Nora tried hard to cover all the differences he was making among the children, and she talked to him about this every day. Nick didn't agree with what she said, but he knew Nora was right.

* * * *

For being only three years old, Sophia was a smart girl, playing with and loving her brother and sister. She spent more time with them than with her mom or dad. She waited for them to come back from school, and then waited quietly for them to finish their homework, so they could play together. Sophia was already good at counting and it seemed that she had the same talent as the rest of her family.

Nora felt very grateful that she'd listened to her sister and kept the baby. It was the best gift she ever gave to Bob and Ana.

Bob was now almost sixteen years old! One day, Nick asked him to go to one of his construction sites. Nick tried to show Nora how much he cared about his children, all his new children. Bob already had a plan. He couldn't take anymore. As soon as he got to the construction site, he tried to stay away from his stepfather's sight. Nick was busy with his construction project, dealing with different workers, giving them directions. He was so busy that he didn't realize Bob wasn't there anymore. Bob had jumped in a bus that took him to a new, unknown life, changing his future forever. Bob was afraid that Nick would try to find him to bring him home. Nick hadn't even noticed Bob's disappearance!

At the end of the day, Nick finally realized Bob wasn't there any longer. He asked everybody around him if somebody saw his stepson. People were so busy doing their own things that nobody had seen the young man. The first thing that came to his mind was Nora.

"Oh my God, she's going to kill me! Where can I find him?

What if he had an accident? What am I going to tell Nora? I'm lost—
I am so lost." He was more afraid of the consequences between Nora
and him, and not really concerned as much for what had happened
to Bob.

* * * *

Bob had no money; he had no place to go. He had no idea where
the bus would take him. He wanted to go back to his mom and his
sisters, but if he went back, his stepfather would be there too. And
that was the last thing he wanted, to be with Nick. Bob decided to
face the world, praying to God to protect him. Not too far from the
construction site, he'd seen a soccer field.

His decision was made in a fraction of a second. He asked the
bus driver to stop and let him get off at the soccer stadium. He
thanked him for letting him ride for free, got off the bus, and went
to the soccer stadium. When he got there, he saw a few soccer
players resting on a bench, drinking water. He said hi and asked if
he could talk to their coach.

Then a man came from the locker room. He stopped in front of
Bob and looked at him, head to toe. He was wondering where this
young man came from.

The neighborhood wasn't populated and it was located outside
of the city. He asked Bob where he came from, where he lived, and
why he wasn't in school, among other questions. The coach was
impressed with Bob's figure, but mostly with the situation, he was
going through. Tim was a good father and he wanted to help this
child, even if he could get in trouble for helping a minor. He let Bob
call his mother to tell her where he was, the address, everything.

Nora screamed at him, "Bob, do not leave that place, please,
stay there! Wait for me. I will come and talk to you. I will come as
soon as I can. Please, do not leave. Put the coach on the phone."

Bob put the coach on the phone, and he heard him say, "Yes,
ma'am; yes, I promise. This is my address. I do not know what kind
of man your son is, or the whole situation, and I hope he will not
leave. He wants to play soccer, but he seems so educated and he

wants to keep going to school."

Tim dictated his address to Ana and when that conversation was over, he said to Bob, "I talked to your mother and I promised her that you would stay at my home till she comes and takes you back home."

"Sir, thank you, but I am not going back home. I love my mother, my sisters and my family, but I cannot live under the same roof with that man anymore. He is a cold man with no feelings. He never abused us, but he never loved us. I feel like a stranger in the house, all the time. I had to run from home. I am so sorry for my mom and my sisters."

"Ok. When this game is over, you can go with me to my home and we'll see what tomorrow will bring."

Tim let Bob hit the ball along the side of the field and he liked what he saw. Bob could become a good soccer player, but he was still so young. School should be his priority, not soccer. When the game was over, the coach approached Bob. "Ok, let's go home now, and thank God, I have a godly wife. She will be happy to take care of you."

Tim was right. When they got to his home and his wife saw him with a young man, she thought he was one of his players. She served them a good dinner and listened to her husband's story about how he met Bob and how his mother would come tomorrow to talk to him.

After Bob went to bed, she mentioned to her husband, "If he doesn't want to go home, maybe it is a sign from God! He could be our son! What do you think? I would love to have a son like him! He is so clean, so pure, and so handsome. He looked like the child I dream of in my dreams. God, let him be ours," she said.

* * * *

Nora took the first train available to get to the address she had. She asked if Maria could take few days off to take care of Ana and Sophia. Maria was more than happy to do so.

The whole family was terrified about what had happened. Nora was blaming herself for letting things go this far, so far that she could lose her own son. Bob was the love of her life; everybody knew it. Bob was her reason to live, to breathe. She would never admit this aloud, saying that she loved her children equally. But Nora knew the truth. She loved him more than she could love anybody, her firstborn. Even her love for Titus was poured over Bob.

Ana was too young to realize this, and she loved her brother so much that she would not even care. Her mom and her brother, her aunt and her cousins, that's all she'd had in her young life. She wanted Nick out of their lives, but he was their mom's husband. Ana begged her mom to bring back Bob, and to not let him live among strangers.

Nora promised to bring him back.

Nora arrived at the coach's house and was greeted by a beautiful, middle-age woman who introduced herself and invited Nora to come in, offering a cup of tea. Nora thanked the woman and asked about her son.

Bob threw himself into his mother's arms.

They cried together, and after a while, Nora asked him, "Why did you do this to me? How could you? What is wrong with you? Why? Why? We need to go home right now."

"Mom, I cannot live in the same place where Nick is. I cannot stand him. I know you, Sophia and Ana need him, but I am not coming back."

"Son, what about school; what about your dream to go to college?"

"I will go to college, but I have to graduate high school first, and I will."

"How?" Nora asked. "How are you going to achieve all this? You're still a very young man. You need your family; we need each other. Let's go home and I will divorce Nick, and we'll find a way to survive. I don't love him. I don't even know why I married him, I don't love him."

"Mom, I don't blame you. You did it for us; you hoped that we were going to have a father to love us, to take care of us, but things didn't go the way you wanted."

"Did he beat you? Did he ever hurt you?"

"No, he didn't, but I feel hurt in a different way. Mom, please, understand me and again, I promise you, I will take care of me and graduate college."

"How are you going to take care of yourself? You are too young to work. You have to be eighteen years old to be accepted. This nice family has no obligations to help you, to feed you. They don't know you; why should they help you?"

"I don't know the answer, but the coach said he would help me."

Nora and Bob agreed to keep in touch with each other, and after talking with the coach and his wife, Nora left, going back to her daughters. She left alone, without the love of her life. She was determined to divorce Nick and live alone with her kids.

Bob then started playing soccer and the coach was pleased to see his talent. He hoped to see Bob become a famous soccer player, but he knew that school had to be the main thing. That family almost adopted Bob. If somebody had asked how this was possible, nobody would have an answer.

Why was that soccer field right there where the bus took Bob? Why did the coach take him under his wings? Nora had all these questions in her mind, all the time. She kept in touch with her son, but her heart was devastated. Bob was her love. Then, she realized she made the same differences as Nick did. How could she say that she loved her son more than everyone else?

But she did. She tried to send him money to help the family with the expenses, but her son was working and going to school.

Bob was doing well and the only thing missing was his family. He came home to visit few times, and he felt like he was recharging his batteries with love, before going back to his new place, to his new family. He graduated high school and started college.

Nora felt grateful to those people for the love they showed to her son. She went for the graduation and felt pride in her son. Bob was handsome and women were paying attention to him. Soon, he met a young woman and he fell in love with her.

He was having the time of his life, but his heart was missing his sisters, his mom, and the whole family.

His sister Sophia was already in elementary school, and she looked like her siblings. She looked nothing like Nick, and this made everybody happy! Though, nobody admitted it.

* * * *

Things were going smoothly; then, one day, Nick came home looking devastated, pale, and frightened.

Even if Nora didn't care much how Nick looked, she noticed the devastation on his face. Something must have happened; something really bad must have happened. "What is wrong with you?" she asked.

"Nora, it is possible I will get fired and be put in jail. Something happened at work. I didn't do anything wrong, but I am responsible for signing some papers. Some people used my signature to steal construction materials, and now the authorities will come after me."

"It is impossible! You didn't steal; somebody else did it."

"I know, but they used my signature."

"Do something. Otherwise, we will have no roof above our heads and no food on the table. With only the money I bring home, we cannot survive."

He nodded and looked so upset. "I wish we had money to hire a lawyer, but even so, the lawyers do what the regime tells them to do. They shouldn't have signed those documents. Nora, I cannot believe what these people did with my papers. I cannot prove that I didn't do anything wrong. I have to find some legal help."

"Ana only has one more year before graduating high school, then she wants to go to college. Ok, I must stop now. We'll see what we can do." Nora wrung her hands.

"Nora, hopefully, everything will be ok. I hope this with all my heart, but we are talking about a huge amount of money, representing the value of those materials. I am done. I am finished. What will happen to you?"

Nora shook her head. "Sophia will need uniforms, a book bag, shoes, and so many other things for school, then with all the bills that come every month. Ana had to insert cardboard in her shoes because they had holes inside. Even with two salaries, we couldn't have a decent life. Can you imagine how we are going to live with one small salary?" Nora asked, but she was mostly talking to herself. She started crying, even though she didn't want to. She felt guilty again, thinking about why she didn't divorce Nick a long time ago.

She knew it was too late to do it now. Nora prayed to God for a miracle. She'd reached the point when she needed a miracle. She couldn't raise her daughters by herself and still be able to go see Bob. She felt grateful Ana had good grades and all her teachers were proud of her. She had the same grades in mathematics and languages, meaning she could go to the math section or the languages section. This meant great things for her future. But Nora realized that Ana had to decide on her own. Whatever she chose would dictate her future. She didn't have any pressure from her teachers or her family. Everybody let her choose what she liked the most. Ana had chosen mathematics, so she was taking physics, mathematics, and chemistry classes in order to go to a good college. Little did she know that her life was about to change forever.

The results from Nick's investigations brought much sorrow and pain to their hearts. Nick's mistake would cost him his freedom for a couple of years. He tried hard to prove that he had good intentions, but the documents had his signature and this had been enough to condemn him. He would go to a special camp, almost like a prison or a work camp. The regime needed healthy men to work on their special projects, their special buildings and Nick was a perfect fit for it.

Nora wouldn't be able to cover the rent, food and all the other bills that keep coming every month. The whole family got together and talked about what needed to be done, so Nora and her daughters could keep the apartment.

Nora ended up getting work in a pastry shop, lifting heavy boxes of bottles filled with water and lemonade all day long. She couldn't find a better job as an accountant's assistant like she had before. Maria and her family tried to help as much as they could, but there wasn't enough for them to cover all the living expenses. The bills were coming, the days were passing by, and the family wasn't able to pay them.

* * * *

Ana had watched all this going on and knew she needed to do something. She told her mom, "Mom, as soon as I graduate high school, I will get a job and help with the bills. We have no money; they are going to throw us into the streets."

"Ana, my dear, we cannot wait till graduation."

"What do you mean? What do you mean we cannot wait?"

"Ana, please, listen to me. It hurts my heart to tell you this. You know how much I love you. We have to do something now, or we will become homeless."

"What can I do? How can I help? I don't get it."

"We have to talk to Peter and ask him to find you a job."

"Do you mean getting a job, at my age? A permanent job? What about my school? I love my school." Ana started crying, realizing that soon she would become an employee, instead of a college student. She looked up and asked God what she did wrong to have such a life at such a young age. Not only had she lost her father, but now she had to give up school for a salary. "Mom, I will do what has to be done. I love you and Sophia with all my heart. I will get a job and go to evening classes like my brother did and hopefully one day, I will graduate college." She hugged her mother and her sister as tears streamed down her face.

Sophia was only seven years old and had no idea why her sister was crying so much. She stared at her mom and she was crying too, so she asked Ana why both of them were crying.

"We have a headache. So let's go and finish your homework, and we can read that story together that you love so much."

"Ok, let's go. I love when you read with me. It feels like I have two moms."

* * * *

Nora looked at her daughters and felt blessings were coming from above. Love would solve everything. She called her nephew Peter who had a good job as a chemical engineer and knew a lot of people. "Hi, Peter, how are you?"

"Oh, Aunt Nora, I am so happy to hear from you, but you don't sound too happy. Are things getting better?"

"No, you know what's happened with Nick, and I know you and Maria tried to help us as much as you could. I am grateful for everything you did for us, but can you stop by after work today? I would like to talk to you."

"Of course, I will be there as soon as I finish my day. See you all soon."

Peter came right after work. He listened to what Nora had to say.

Nora explained to her nephew that Ana has to work and bring home a salary in order to keep living in the apartment.

Peter looked at his cousin, Ana and he couldn't stop thinking how beautiful and sad she was.

Peter found himself thinking, she is my sister, we grew up together, and I need to help her. He was determined to find a job for Ana. He promised to do his best. As soon as he got to work, the very next morning, he would go to his boss and explain the situation.

* * * *

While her mother and cousin discussed her future, Ana realized her dreams were ruined. All the people she knew had their children living at home and going to school.

Her brother chose to run away from home and God helped him to find his way in life. But it was a different situation…he was a man…she was a girl. All her classmates would finish high school and have graduation together; she would be at work.

It didn't take Peter long to call with good news; he found a job for Ana. Nora had to go to the City Hall and ask for a waiver, because of Ana's age. She was only two months short of being eighteen years old, which was the legal working age.

Escape

Ana's mind was busy. When her cousin called and told them the news, she became anxious about her job—her first job! How would it be? What would she do there and what kind of job would it be? Ana had so many questions. So, she prayed that things would go smoothly and that people would teach her how to do things right.

She had a job interview that went really well, but Ana noticed how the man treated her like a child. He even told her he had children her age. Ana drew the conclusion that his children were going to school, not to work. But she was determined to help her family. Her dreams had to wait. She signed a few papers and was told she would start in a week.

Ana realized she didn't have dresses or outfits for work. Being in school, she was wearing uniforms, saving them lots of money. Her mom and her aunt modified some of their clothes and made them pretty, so Ana would feel comfortable among the new people she would meet at work.

When Ana started going to work, she enjoyed everybody she met. There were good people, willing to teach her and show her how to do things. Her training went wonderfully.

Peter couldn't have been more proud of her. People congratulated him for having such a smart and beautiful relative. Ana brought a fresh air to her work place, a "young blood" they had never had before.

She was placed in the blueprint drafting department where she learned how to calculate objects' weight and how to draw sections through the metal parts for chemical equipment. She loved it and became really good at it. Ana was promoted and very much appreciated. She brought home every penny she earned.

One day, even though she knew her mom would argue with her for spending money, she brought home a large bouquet of flowers. She knew what flowers meant for her mom.

Nora was in tears when she saw the flowers. It had been such a long time since she received flowers. Memories came to her mind, but she knew it was not the right moment. Being poor didn't allow her to dream. She hugged her daughter and didn't even argue about the money spent. Nora had been too happy to receive them.

"Thank you, thank you, my dear! I love those flowers. Thank you." She arranged the flowers in a nice crystal vase that had been made by Titus and remembered the good times.

There were so many things needing to be done.

Ana enrolled in evening classes and eventually lost contact with her high school friends. She had no time for friendship. She had to work, study to graduate, and then go to college. Between Ana and her friends, their activities now were so different, and she always had a question in the back of her mind. *Why am I so different than my friends? Why is my life so hard? Why did I lose my father? Why did my mother have to marry that man? Why did my brother have to run away from home? Why did I have to give up school and work? Why? Why?*

She realized her entire life was wrapped up in those questions, and only God had the answers. Ana knew this, and she let things roll the way her fate decided, but she was still determined to finish school.

* * * *

When Nick came back home from the disciplinary camp, he got a job that paid a lot less than he had before, but it was a job. He didn't stay long there, but long enough to change Ana's life forever. Ana didn't blame him for her fate; she blamed him more for not being a "normal" father, who cared about his children, who loved them. She didn't ask for more, but it would be so nice to have somebody asking you how your day went. How you felt, if you were ok or not, just minor unimportant questions, but so important to have your father ask you. The only human being in his world was Sophia.

Nora and Nick had so many divergences that they were spending their lives like two strangers. Nora had no eyes for her husband and she had no feelings for him. All her hopes to have a loving family were gone. Her family was her children, her sister, and her sister's family. In her mind, she had no husband.

Ana was happy to see her younger sister. They had dinner, and looking at Sophia, she remembered how much time they spent with

Bob and how wonderful that time was.

"Mom, let's go and see Bob. Sophia can go too."

"Don't say this, please. You know how much I miss him. There is no way we can afford to go. It will cost so much. We just have enough to cover our expenses. My God, how much I would love to be with him, to hold him tight. We live in tough times, Ana, and my heart cries for all of us. Thank you again, for the beautiful flowers. Good night and God take care of you. You are my angel!"

"Good night, Mom, you have three angels."

The next day at work, Ana's boss gave her a paper and said, "Ana, please fill out this form as soon as possible, and when you are done, return it back to me. Thank you."

"Yes, sir, I will." She looked at the paper and said, "Again?"

"What do you mean 'again'?" her boss asked.

"I returned this form last month."

"Oh, so you already enrolled in our Party?"

"No, sir, I cannot enroll now, because I am attending evening school and during the day, I am here at work. Six days a week at work and school is also six evenings a week. There is no time for me to be active and participate at all those meetings."

"You are right, those meetings are weekly and it takes a lot of time. But nobody can be excused from becoming a member. I will try my best, but you have to take it in consideration. There is no other option. Everybody has to be a member of the Communist Party; it is their rule. One of them," he said and left the office where Ana worked.

Ana knew there were things left untold during their conversation. Her boss was a very educated, smart man and he was treating everybody with respect. She knew he hated the new regime as much as she did, but nobody dared to talk about it. It was a very dangerous thing to say what you think or to comment about it.

Ana's boss knew exactly why she refused to sign the application. He didn't want to do it either, but he had to. He had to be a good example for his employees, for the workers under his supervision.

Ana's colleagues were in love with her attitude, her

selflessness, and her smile. And even on her birthday, when she came to work, people sang to her, brought flowers and chocolate then all day long, she was their princess.

"How did you know it was my birthday? I almost forgot about it. Oh, it must have been Peter, my cousin, he told you. Thank you so much for being such good people. You taught me many things, and I love all of you. Ok, I will make a strong Turkish coffee for everybody. You've made me feel so appreciated, so happy. Thank you." All this joy and appreciation made her wonder why she didn't feel the same way at home, with her stepfather.

CHAPTER NINE

One day, a coworker invited Ana to have lunch together. It seemed innocent enough when he clarified that they could eat here at the work place, not go out. He was a tall, handsome man, thin and quiet. They'd never exchanged more than everyday greetings, but they seemed to like each other.

"Ana, I see you every day, but I've never had the nerve to ask you out. I am glad to have lunch with you."

"I am glad too."

They didn't need too many words to feel comfortable with each other. Then the next day, he asked her again to share lunch together; she gladly accepted. His name was Steven.

"So, what kind of work do you do here, Steven?"

"Oh, you don't know? I thought you knew what department I worked in."

"I know where you work, but I was never that curious to find out the name of the department."

"It is a chemical lab where we test all the probes for rubber before going into fabrication."

"I see; do you like it?"

"Actually, I love it. It is so interesting, the work I do. Time flies by quickly. What about you?"

"I love what I do, but I don't think I will do this forever. I work in the blueprint department, and I learned a lot about how to take a piece of equipment, our type of equipment, measure it, cross-section it, make it three-dimensional, plus standard writing. I use a large drawing board to draw it. But I am interested in beauty products."

Ana realized she'd never talked so much. She was really comfortable in Steven's presence. He always seemed so calm, and she was all over the place, full of energy!

"Like what?" Steven asked. "What kind of beauty products do you feel interested in?"

"I often see my mom saving egg whites, mixing them with lemon, sometimes with honey, and put it on her face. The first time I saw her doing this, I laughed, but when she applied it on me, I liked it. I loved it. I would like to make people happy and to make them look better. I like people."

"Are you happy, Ana?"

His question caught her off-guard. It was the last thing she expected to hear from his mouth. "Why do you ask me such a question?"

"Because of your eyes. They look sad to me."

"Oh no, I am happy. I am as happy as I can be," Ana said with a few tears in her eyes. Steven knew she wasn't happy; he could read her face. He wished he could make her happy, to see her really happy. Her smile was amazing, but something seemed to be missing. He realized he was in love with Ana.

* * * *

A few months went by, and Steven invited Ana to a friend's birthday party, but she refused to go. She never liked parties, considering them a waste of time. She preferred to read a good book. She remembered how many times she read *Gone with the Wind*. She even knew entire pages by heart. Five times, she'd read that book, and it wasn't enough. A good book was taking her away from the present, taking her to places where she would never go; a good book was Ana's best friend.

Steven was shocked to hear her refusal, but he respected her wish.

Ana told her mom about Steven's invitation and the fact that she said no. "Why don't you go? You stay home all the time. Go and have fun. You work together, you know who he is, and you told me he's a gentleman. Go, dance and have fun. Life is not just work, work, and more work." She kissed Ana and started focusing on her own stuff; she had plenty to do.

So, Ana contacted Steven. "Steven, I changed my mind. If you still want me to go with you, I will."

Steven was dancing on the clouds, feeling happy and lucky.

Sophia and Nora were fixing the last details on Ana's dress. Sophia looked up at her sister, grabbed her hand, and said, "You are so beautiful. I want to be as beautiful as you are when I grow up. I love you, sis!"

"You will be even more beautiful than you think I am. Just wait. You are already a beauty." Then, Ana looked over at her mom and said, "Mom, you know, all women wear those pantyhose with black line on the back. I don't have them, but if you give me your black eyeliner, I can draw a line so it will look like I have them on! And I will not sit down, so it will stay put."

Everybody was speechless.

"How are going to do it?"

"You know I draw things. I can do it."

"Oh my God, only you could come with such an idea. It is genius. Do you see what poverty is teaching us? No, I take my words back. We aren't poor, even though we cannot afford to have fancy things."

Nora gave Ana her eyeliner and she couldn't believe the perfection of the line Ana drew on the back of her legs. It looked like she had those pantyhose on! It looked so elegant and sophisticated. "Ana, I'm so proud of the woman you have become: smart, intelligent, and very beautiful. I hope your sister will be the same when she gets older. Enjoy your time and don't worry about anything. It is your time; put all your heart in it."

Ana was ready to meet Steven and go to his friend's birthday party. She felt nervous. It was the first time she would be going somewhere by herself without family.

* * * *

Steven had always thought Ana was beautiful, but when he came to pick her up from her apartment, he couldn't talk. He thought she was the most beautiful girl in the world, and he asked himself how he got so lucky to go out with such a beauty. Her cat eyes, her black hair, her body was thin but curvy. "And, this girl likes me?"

They arrived at Steven's friend's house and people were already dancing and laughing, having fun. Steven introduced Ana to everybody, and she received lots of compliments, even from the other girls. They were about the same age and had things in common.

Ana felt good and comfortable, like she'd known them forever. A young man came and asked Ana to dance with him, but for some reason she said no. She danced with Steven, and she enjoyed each moment of the party, like her mom wished for her.

After a while, the same young man approached Ana and said, "May I have a dance with you, please? I already asked Steven's permission."

She smiled and was tempted to say he didn't have to ask Steven's permission, but she didn't say one word about it. "Yes, let's dance." Steven's friend touched Ana's hand, leading her to the dance floor, a small space already filled with young couples. The moment he touched her hand, the sky sent lighting and thunder over Ana's body. Taken by surprise, she removed her hand and stopped for a second. *What is happening to me? What did I just feel?* She made an effort to go back to 'normal' and started dancing with this young man without to even knowing his name. She remembered he'd introduced himself, but she hadn't paid attention.

When the music was over, he took her back to Steven, kissed her hand, and said, "Thank you for dancing with me. I will remember this dance forever."

Ana didn't say one word and remained kind of quiet for the rest of the party.

Steven seemed to feel like he was the happiest person on earth. He took Ana back to her apartment, kissed her hand and wished her good night.

When Ana got home, her mom was waiting for her, to be sure

she got home safe.

She looked at her daughter and asked her if she had fun and enjoyed the party. "Oh, Mom, it was wonderful. I danced and danced," she said, and while she talked, she twirled as if she were back on that dance floor.

"I am glad. You haven't had any chance ever to go to a party. I am afraid I was too strict."

"How can you say you have been too strict? Oh, no!" Ana was joking, knowing the truth. Her mom was very strict, but everybody was like this, especially parents that had girls. "I love you, Mom, but I like to be with people too. Let's go to bed. We have to be ready for tomorrow."

* * * *

Ana loved taking care of Sophia, being the big sister, the teacher, the caregiver, everything. Nothing could separate them, even Ana's stepfather. He was actually happy to see how much Sophia loved Ana, but with his nature, he could not show his feelings.

Ana looked around the small apartment. *I wish I could escape this place, to run away like my brother did. Of course, I can but what about my little sister and my mom? They are my world they are everything to me. I cannot do that to them. I have to stay here with them and God will help me find a way. We're healthy and we love each other, except for my stepfather.*

Bob came to visit his family and introduce his future wife. What a joy! The whole family got together, Maria, John, Peter, and Chris, looking like a gathering from the old days when they spent time with one another. Everybody loved Bob's fiancée; she had amazing blue eyes and short red hair. It was so easy to see how much they loved each other.

Nora was happy to see her son and how much he had grown into a man, getting married and ready to start a family. When she realized how much her son loved his fiancée, acceptance of her future daughter-in-law was easy. She knew her son came to get her blessing and that he didn't need her acceptance to marry his fiancée, but it was a mother-son thing, full of respect and love.

Ana couldn't take her eyes from her brother and his love. She felt like she wanted to leave and be with them. But again, her sister and her mom were her obligation, her duty and love. She had to stay with them until she got married. For one moment, her thoughts were stronger than her heart, but she came back to reality. "Bob, I am so happy for you. Adie is adorable; she will be my best friend. Now I have two sisters; thank you, brother."

"Thank you, sister. I'm in love with Adie. I want to take care of her till the end of my life. I know we live in tough times, but I want kids, at least one."

"Oh, this is good for you! I want kids too, but I have to get married first!" Ana laughed, even while she hoped the day would come.

"I have no worries about you getting married! The man that marries you will be the luckiest on Earth, and I say this with all my heart. I love you, sister. I want to live closer to you and our family, especially Sophia. I would like to be a bigger part of her education and to help our mom more. Do you remember when Sophia was in a stroller and you and I were pushing the stroller down the street, our windy street? My God, we were so lucky we didn't kill her or put her into the hospital with major injuries. When I look back at how we played with her, I know only God saved us and her. The street had been too steep, and the stroller was way faster than us. He was watching over us. He knew how much we wanted her to have fun and how much we enjoyed playing with her. I love Sophia, but her father? How can I carry his last name? I want to change it back to our own father's last name, but that would create friction between Mom and him and I cannot see our mom suffering. I will wait and maybe later on, I will change my last name."

Brother and sister had a long-needed conversation…two souls were getting their wounds opened to heal.

"Bob, I'm not happy and you know this. I wanted to run away like you did, but I couldn't do this to my mom—our mom and to Sophia. They need me so much. My dreams are gone. I go to work and evening school, and that is it. Thank God, a friend of mine, a coworker, invited me to a party and I was able to see that life isn't only about work and work."

"Sister, do not ever think about leaving the family. It is different for a man than for a woman. People can take advantage of you. You are so young and beautiful. I know you're smart, but being smart is not enough to survive in this 'jungle' called the world, called life. Stay home and I promise I will visit more often, to help you and Mom as much as I can. I will graduate college and get a good job with a good salary. Promise me that you won't make a wrong move."

"Don't worry, you know better. I wouldn't leave my mom and my sister. I'm almost her mother that is how much I love her. Whatever I spoke with you, you're the only one who knows what is in my mind and heart."

"Now I feel a lot better. You scared me for a moment. I think I came at the right moment. I came to introduce Adie to all of you, but it seems that it was the right time to talk to you. I'm so glad I came. Let's go and join the 'tribe'! Oh, I forgot to tell you that I hope to become a soccer coach later on. I love soccer so much, but I love what I'm studying now too. I will graduate with a degree in history and geography, and I may become a teacher. We'll see. One way or the other, I will teach and play soccer. Not bad for somebody that ran away from home at sixteen years old!"

* * * *

Adie met all the family members, enjoying each moment. She could feel everything Bob told her was so true. Nora was like a sister, like an older sister, protecting her and showing her affection. Maria was like an old friend that she had known forever. Sophia stood next to her all the time. The cousins were just so friendly that she couldn't believe how lucky she was to enter such a good family.

Adie had been nervous and shy when she was introduced to Bob's family, but now she was laughing and talking to everybody like she'd been part of the family since she was born.

She looked at Bob with gratitude and love. He was talking to his sister, Ana but he smiled at her, making her feel really happy. *What a family and what kind people! My family is a lot different; it would take them a while to treat a stranger like Bob's family treated me.* Adie already felt a part of the big family and she couldn't wait to come back, to visit. Or for them to come and visit after she and Bob got married. They said goodbye and went back to their home to get ready for the wedding. It was their happy time, full of hopes and dreams.

Ana knew how much joy Bob's visit brought for her mom. Nora's eyes were like fireworks; she smiled all day long and looked years younger. It never bothered Ana that her mom loved Bob more than she loved anybody else. He was and would remain her favorite, her firstborn, the boy! Nora never admitted this out loud, but everybody knew the truth: she loved her son more than her own eyes, and seeing him happy was making her even happier. It was just another "mother thing."

Ana cleaned up the room and went to bed thanking God for having them all, and she even mentioned Nick in her prayers.

* * * *

The end of fall came with beautiful sunsets, linden tree leaves and dried flowers covering the streets. Ana loved those linden trees. When she was younger, her mom used to take her and Bob for a walk under those amazing trees. The fragrance of the flowers brought to mind beautiful memories full of images she would never forget. She thought there was something special about how she associated those happy images with that fragrance, the smell that brought back memories.

Looking at her mom and the things she was doing, those beautiful images went away. Nora was trying to make some winter provisions. It was so different from how her grandparents used to make those. That was a long, long time ago. They used to have a long, huge, deep basement with shelves to store smoked meats, root vegetables, fruits, wine, brandy, and flour, almost everything they needed to survive the heavy winters.

Now, they had a tiny apartment with an open balcony. Nora tried to improvise a way to store some necessary things for the times when they couldn't get out in a storm or the heavy, high snow. There were days when they weren't able to open the apartment building door because it was blocked by snow.

Ana remembered those times and it made her feel stronger.

She also remembered, *"We do as much as we can with what we have."* What she'd learned from her mom and her aunt when they had to make things with whatever they could find. She knew how to make surrogate coffee from some beans, how to make cottage cheese using lemon, and a lot more. The need, basic necessity, made them all creative and in the end, this was something good. The Communist Party put the country in a survival mode and made people get creative.

Christmas was getting closer and it was a big holiday for the whole country. Even if people didn't have the means to buy presents and bake all the good holiday favorites, you could still see how much they enjoyed the preparation, the decoration of their homes or apartments, doing the best they could.

An amazing aroma was in the air, all the homes smelled like the holidays. If somebody asked where they had the money to buy all these things, the answer would be a lift of their shoulders. Nobody knew the answer, but they had a minimum of food, wine, and goods on their tables.

God always provided for his people. Ana and her family were huge believers in this miracle, being grateful.

Ana's coworker and friend, Steven, invited her out again, to go to a Christmas party. The party was few days before Christmas; otherwise, she would never have accepted the invite if it meant leaving her family alone on Christmas day. Ana was glad to go to the party, but she wasn't so sure she wanted to spend all the time with Steven. She hoped to see that man again and dance with him.

"Ana, I received orders to go to the army, for service. All men have to go to the army when they reach a certain age. So, my turn is getting closer, and I have only one regret that I didn't get to know you better. I love you, Ana!"

Ana didn't at all expect to hear these words from Steven. She didn't do anything to be loved. She considered herself to be a good friend, nothing more than that. Her heart stopped for a moment, but she kept walking, avoiding Steven's eyes.

He knew there would be no answer. He knew she would never love him. "I know you don't like parties, but sometimes you need to forget about your own problems and like you said, take it like a medicine."

"Steven, I am sorry you have to go to the army. Thank you for being a good friend."

"I am going to miss you, Ana. You made my life sunnier. I love spending time with you. I cannot wait to see you in the morning when I come to work. I hope you will still spend some time with me when I come back."

"How long are you going to be gone? Oh, I remember—you said six months. The time will fly and you will be back fast."

"Before I met you, six months meant nothing to me, but now it will feel like eternity," Steven said.

Ana put her head down and kept walking next to Steven.

Both of them left the conversation blank.

Ana was dressed in a simple skirt and a sweater, but Steven looked at her like he was seeing her for the first time. "Ana, you look very nice. Simple... I like it."

"Oh, this is what I was wearing today at work. Do you think it will be ok to be dressed like this, or do I have to go home and change my clothes? Actually, I don't have too many clothes to change into."

"No, don't do that. You look beautiful. I love your outfit, and I love you!"

"Thank you, Steven. By the way, you look really good. It seems like you spent your entire salary on you." She laughed.

"Actually, I do. My sister is married, and she has her own family. My parents are gone, and I am alone. It is only me to take care of. There is nobody else."

"I heard from my colleagues that there is an older lady that works with you, and she adores you. I am happy for you."

"Don't be happy for me. She might adore me, but I love you," he said.

Ana wanted to slap herself on the mouth. Why did she have to mention that people talk about Steven? Now he would think she cared about him, when she didn't…not in that way. She only thought of him as a good friend, and hoped he was smart enough to see it.

When Ana and Steven arrived at the party, Steven rang the bell and a young man opened the door.

It was Alex. Ana remembered his name, from when he'd mentioned it at the birthday party, and for the first time in her life, she felt butterflies in her stomach. She had no idea why they called it butterflies, but that's how she felt. "Hi, how are you?" she greeted the young man with a smile and a handshake.

"Hi, Ana. I am Alex. Do you remember me?" He took her hand and very politely, kissed it.

"Kind of? Oh, wait a minute! We danced together; now I remember," she said. She had remembered very well, but wouldn't let him know this.

Steven hugged his friend and greeted everybody.

Ana joined a group of young women that were sitting on the chairs, talking about life, men, and children, among other things. Later on, she would never remember what they all talked about. Her eyes followed Alex everywhere he went, paying attention to what he was doing. When Alex invited one of those young women to dance with him, Ana felt a sharp thorn hurting her heart. She was so mad at herself for it too. *I don't even know him, not even his full name—forget about knowing him as a person, and I am already jealous?*

She stopped looking at him and tried to get more involved in the conversation she was having with the other young ladies.

Steven and Alex came closer to the group, apologized for interrupting their conversation, and asked Ana to join them.

Curious, Ana excused herself and came closer to Steven. "Well," she asked. "Where's the fire? This seems so urgent."

"Ana, do you remember my friend Alex? I asked him to take you out when you feel like you want to have fun, so you will have somebody trustworthy. Of course, only if you agree with this. If not, at least I tried to leave you in good hands. You don't have to answer now. I just want to see if you like the idea."

This surprised her a lot. "Thank you, Steven. I will think about it. And thank you, Alex."

"May I give Alex your phone number, so he can check on you?"

"Yes, thank you."

Later that evening, Alex invited Ana to dance with him.

The world was spinning for Ana. His touch, his body, his moves, everything screamed love! She tried to hide the way she felt, but she knew Steven saw right away that she would never be his.

He didn't say a word all evening. He took Ana back to her apartment, kissed her on her cheeks, and said, "Thank you, Ana, for coming with me to the party. I will see you tomorrow." He hesitated, then spoke again slowly. "I love you," he tried once more.

"Thank you, good night, and see you tomorrow at work."

Ana was so transformed, smiling the entire way upstairs to the last floor where she lived.

Nora was waiting for her to be sure she got home and to say good night. And because a mother didn't miss one thing about her children, she noticed how happy Ana looked. "Ana, I'm so happy you had such a good time. It shows on your face. Your eyes look happy. I haven't seen you like this for a long time."

"Mom, I'm in love. I don't know him well, but I am in love with him."

"What are you talking about? You don't even know what love is!"

"You're right, but I love him. I will get to know him when the time comes."

Ana's mother shook her head, even though her heart and her mind were happy thinking that her daughter had found love. She remembered how she felt when her eyes met Titus's eyes. Butterflies, thunder, lightning, all at the same time! She looked up and thanked God for what just happened. "God, thank you. Ana is in your hands now; bless her with your gifts, like you blessed me." Nora slept better than ever.

* * * *

Ana woke up happy and ready to go to work. People around her noticed her glow. The day went by like she wasn't there, but she did all her work with so much exuberance and pleasure that some of her coworkers asked her what was her secret. She answered by smiling. It was a pleasure to be around her; she was loved so much by all her coworkers.

"Ana, Sophia, dinner is ready," Nora said.

"Thank you, Mom, but I'm not hungry," Ana said, sitting next to her sister.

"You are so pale! Are you sick? Where is your smile? Is something wrong at work? Tell me, please."

"No, the work is fine. Actually, I got promoted, so more money for all of us."

"Oh, thank God. So, why are you so sad?"

Sophia was all ears, not being able to understand what was going on with her sister that she loved so much.

Nora realized that Ana couldn't talk in Sophia's presence, so she said, "Let's eat. The food is getting cold."

As soon as they finished dinner, Ana cleaned up and put things where they belonged. Nora waited until Sophia went to bed and asked her daughter to open up and tell her what was on her mind. She couldn't stand to see Ana sad. "Ana, please, talk to me. Are you pregnant?"

"Mom, how can you ask such a thing? You know better than everybody I don't go out with anybody. I am not married. How could I be pregnant?"

"I know it, but what makes you so sad?"

"Mom, it is Alex. That's his name. He was supposed to call and check on me while our friend Steven is gone in the army. Alex hasn't called, not even once."

"Did you call him?"

"Me? Over my dead body! I would never call him first. You taught me that a woman has to be chased. But this isn't about being chased or not. I just think he forgot about me, and this bothers me."

"Nobody could forget about you, Ana. You are too precious, and I am sure he feels the same way about you. Believe me, he is in love and scared of what he feels. He is young, too. Give him time to wake up from dreaming of you."

"Maybe I am precious in your eyes…you are my mom! But thank you, Mom. You know what? Let's forget about this and what will be, will be! Night is a good adviser as Aunt Maria always says. I love you, thank you for talking to me. I needed you, and you made me feel better. Good night."

* * * *

On the other side of Bucharest, in a modest house with a beautiful yard, Alex was lost in his thoughts. Every single second of the day, he'd wanted to call Ana and he had to stop his instincts to pick up the phone and dial the number. He didn't want to look desperate, but he was feeling that way. He couldn't stop thinking about her.

"My God, her eyes, her skin! The way she talks, her humor, the way she walks! That's all I have in my mind. I cannot study like I did before, and the finals are getting closer! I have to concentrate on school. I have a few more months till graduation! My mind has no peace. I have to hear her voice, at least to talk to her—my God, I am in love and do not even know her well. What if she doesn't care about me? No, that isn't possible. I feel like she does care about me; she likes me. Okay, I'll just call her, so at least I can find out if she even remembers me."

He picked up the phone and dialed Ana's number, at least to hear her voice. Ana's mother answered the phone, and with a very polite tone, Alex introduced himself and asked if he could talk to Ana.

"Of course, wait a minute, Alex," she said and brought her daughter to the phone.

"Thank you, ma'am, thank you," Alex kept saying.

"Hello?" Ana said.

"Hi, Ana, it is me Alex. How are you? How are you doing?"

"Oh, thank you for calling. I am doing really well—thank you. What about you? How's school?"

Alex started talking about his classes and how busy he was studying because finals and graduation were getting closer. "Since the last time I saw you, my life has only been school and home. I didn't meet one friend and I haven't even seen a movie. Would you like to see a movie with me? You would do me a huge favor by saying yes."

"Do you need a break from studying? I would be happy to help you, but is this the only reason?" Ana found herself asking what she never wanted to ask. This would show him her feelings. I am so stupid, she scolded herself.

"No, it isn't the only reason. Steven asked me to check on you, but I found that I want to be with you," Alex admitted, barely breathing.

"Alex, I would like to go with you to the movie, but not today. Can we plan for Saturday afternoon?" Ana was so mad over what she said to Alex, that she tried to fix her mistake.

Alex was thrilled to get a yes from Ana and any day was ok with him, just to see her. "Of course, Saturday afternoon is perfect. I will be happy to pick you up from your home, if you give me the address. This way your parents can see me," Alex answered in a heartbeat, without thinking too much.

"Oh no, tell me where to meet you, and I will come directly from work. I work Saturday, every Saturday."

"I didn't know you worked, but that is perfect. Let me know where you want to meet, and I will be there waiting for you."

"Wait for me? Are you so sure I will be late?"

"No, but I want to wait for you. I'm so happy to do so."

They agreed on the place to meet and ended the call.

* * * *

Ana felt so happy, she danced a happy dance all over their tiny living room, singing, smiling. She couldn't wait to see Alex.

Sophia was doing her homework, and when she saw her sister

dancing, she jumped from her chair and joined her. How happy they were. Sophia had no idea why her sister was dancing, but if her sister was happy, she was happy too.

Nora came home from work and she saw her daughters dancing and laughing, and her heart filled with happiness. She hugged them both and asked, "Sophia, did you finish your homework? Ana, you look so good." Nora put her hand up to her ear, looking like a phone, and asked silently how "the call" went.

Ana nodded, and then there were three happy people dancing in that tiny living room.

When Nora and Ana were finally alone, Nora asked about the call from Alex.

"He had to study for finals. Oh, I didn't tell you that he will graduate college in a few months."

"I am glad he goes to college; this is a good sign."

"So, what does that mean? If I am not going to college, I am not a 'good sign'?"

"Oh no, dear. We all know how many qualities you have. I didn't mean it that way. You will be in college too, hopefully soon." Nora tried to change the conversation.

Ana had an open wound in her heart…college. She knew she was smart and diligent and better than most of the girls her age. She knew how important college would be for her future. Her cousins had graduated college. Chris was going to the law school and Peter was already a big boss. Her brother put himself through college, and most of her family members had a higher education, except her. "One day, I will," she said out loud. "One day, I will go to college." She helped her mom get things ready, so they could go to bed. She kissed her mom and said, "Mom, I know you didn't want to hurt me! One day, I will go to college, I promise. Good night." She knew her mom would have no rest thinking that she hurt Ana with what she said about college, so Ana showed her she wasn't upset by it.

* * * *

The day came when Ana and Alex met to go and see a movie.

She arrived on time and saw Alex waiting for her. He was all put together: his tie and shirt had beautiful colors, and his shoes were shining.

I cannot believe I am looking at his shoes, when the only thing I want is to get lost in his eyes. Am I crazy? She kept looking down so Alex wouldn't see her happiness, her joy. Ana felt so happy to be with Alex, to talk to him, to walk next to him, just to be together.

When the movie was over, Alex asked if she wanted to have something sweet, an ice cream…something so they could sit down and talk, to spend more time with together.

Ana accepted his invitation and they walked and talked all the way to the small coffee shop.

It was crowded, especially after the movie, because everybody was going there. They found a small table in the corner of the coffee shop and enjoyed being together, getting to know each other, sharing things, laughing. It felt like they were alone with no other people around them. Alex and Ana were in their own world, the world of love.

Alex took Ana to her apartment and asked if he could call again.

"Of course, anytime. Good night."

Nora was waiting for her daughter to get back. When Ana opened the door, she knew that it was love for sure. Now, she could go to bed and pray for God's mercy.

CHAPTER TEN

"Ana, I would like to see you in my office," her boss said.

"Yes, sir, I will be there in a second." She thought maybe she'd done something wrong, but she couldn't remember doing anything like that. So, she went to her boss's office feeling nervous.

"Ana, you are one of the best employees we have and you are among the few that isn't a member of the Communist Party. I don't think I can excuse you anymore. Not being a member will stop your future promotions. You deserve a higher salary; you are so smart."

"I know, sir, how much you have tried to excuse me, and I am grateful for this. Thank you very much. I will see what I can do. I see people losing their jobs for refusing to become members. I have to keep my job. I love my job. And I know I can talk to you… I don't want to become a member of this party. My father lost his life because of the new regime. He couldn't take it anymore and he took his own life."

"I am so sorry to hear this. Peter told me something about that a long time ago. I'm really sorry. I understand more than you think. Let me see what I can do for you. By the way, our director wants you to go to a high technical school where you can get a higher-level diploma. It's a great honor and a huge opportunity. There are people that started work at the same time as you and they were not chosen. I am proud of you."

"Thank you sir, for saying this. Of course, I will go to any school you send me to, but I still have to work. My family needs my salary."

"Do not worry, you will get paid to go to school, so maybe the new regime is not so bad," her boss whispered so nobody could hear. Ana's boss knew her situation. He had wondered why such a smart girl like her didn't go to college, why she had chosen to work, but that was before he found out about the tragedy. It was clearly a tragedy that had changed her life.

Ana's mind was running miles per second. She wondered if going to school would keep her from seeing Alex, but she always had faith in God that he would make things happen.

The day had been beautiful and now the sunset was just magnificent. Thinking about her promotion at work and the possibility of more education put her in a good mood, despite her worries.

Then, Alex called and asked Ana if she would like to have dinner with his family in the yard, enjoying the sunset.

"Alex, are you sure? I don't know. I don't know anybody!"

"You know me. Don't worry; they will be happy to meet you."

"Well, I'm not sure, but if you say so—I will go."

Alex brought Ana to his family's house. He had two wonderful sisters and living at the same address, an aunt with her family. Ana was shocked by the similarity. Her family used to live like this: one sister and her family on one side of the yard, and another sister with her family on the other side! What an amazing coincidence. It took Ana only a couple of minutes to feel comfortable and welcomed.

Alex's sisters were very friendly, just a few years older than Alex. He was their baby brother, the only brother, and they adored him. Alex's mother was so attentive, making sure there was lots of food on the table for Ana to eat. The time she spent with Alex's family that night reminded her the good old times, when her family could spend time together. Alex's father was exactly what a father should look and behave like. Warm and kind with a big smile on his face, he enjoyed a glass of wine and the good food. His good mood was contagious.

Alex's mother was busy preparing food, and Ana realized she could use some help. "Let me do it, ma'am," Ana asked to help her.

"Oh, call me Stephanie. I am glad you came. It is the first time Alex has brought a girl home, and I am happy that girl is you."

Ana had a response, but she kept it to herself... *and the last girl?* Then she couldn't help but think... *Am I crazy again? Do I expect him to marry me? He doesn't even know me well, and I'm not even sure I would like to marry him.*

They spent an excellent time together, feeling like they knew each other forever.

What a wonderful feeling; what a nice family.

After a while, Ana excused herself, saying it was getting late and she had to go home.

* * * *

Alex took her home, thanking her for accepting his invitation to spend time with his family. Saying good night, he lifted Ana's chin and looked deep into her eyes.

He just wanted to fill his heart with the image of her face, to keep in his memory, to feel her closer to him when he was alone.

Everybody liked Ana; she seemed to be comfortable with my family. I heard the most wonderful things about her, and I want to spend all my time with her. I love being with this smart girl. I want to marry her. If I wait, Ana could find somebody else to marry. Her age is perfect for marriage. I don't want to lose her. I want her to be my wife. How am I going to provide for the family? I have to wait. Alex's mind was so busy with this silent dialogue that he didn't hear Ana's question.

Everything happened when he looked into her eyes. "Ana, I'm so sorry. I didn't hear your question."

"I asked if you're okay. You seemed to be troubled."

"Oh no, I just have too much on my mind, mostly about us."

"What do you mean 'us'?"

"Ana, will you be my wife?"

Thunder couldn't have done more to shock Ana than Alex's question did! "Did you ask me to be your wife? Did I understand it right? Alex, you don't even know me well enough, it takes time to know somebody."

"You're right, but I do know you well enough to know that I

want to be with you for the rest of my life. I know I'm young, but we are the same age. And what I feel for you, I know it is only once in a lifetime. I would be honored to have you as my wife. Ana, I love you with all my heart and my entire mind."

They stopped in the middle of the street.

Ana couldn't breathe; it was so unexpected. Not in a million years did she expect to hear that question. She wasn't ready to say yes or no—the only thing she knew was what her heart told her, and she said it out loud, "Yes, I want to marry you, to be your wife."

He lifted her from the ground and spun around with her in his arms. "Thank you, thank you! I love you."

"Oh God, my mom! I have to tell her first."

"Me too, my parents will be shocked. Let's get together tomorrow and start making plans. We have no money, but we have each other!" Alex took her all the way to the apartment door, kissed her with passion, and flew down the stairs. When he got home, everybody was already sleeping except his mom.

She always waited for her son with warm food. Because Alex was young and very active, playing sports, he was hungry all the time.

"Mom, sit down and get ready to listen to this: I am getting married. I found my bride."

"What are you talking about? What bride?"

"Ana, she will be my bride."

"What about college, army, job?"

"I promise you, everything will be done the way it is supposed to be done."

"Are you serious or this is a joke?"

"Mom, this is not a joke. I want to marry Ana before I graduate college. Actually, there are only three more months and I will be done with school."

"Son, where are you going to live? Ok, I have so many questions—I better go to sleep and we'll continue the conversation tomorrow. I still believe you're joking. Good night, son, I love you."

* * * *

Ana's mom was tired that day so she couldn't wait for Ana to get home like she usually did. She trusted her daughter, so she went to bed to get some sleep. She was exhausted from the heavy lifting and standing all day long.

Nora woke up early in the morning to get Sophia ready for school and have her precious time with Ana, chatting about everything. But Ana was sleeping late because she had an important seminar at work around 2:00 p.m., so Nora let her sleep in.

Suddenly, she noticed a piece of paper on the table. She must have been too busy to notice it before. Nora looked at and almost fainted.

Ana had written the note: *Mom, I am getting married. I love Alex. Love you all.*

She went to the bathroom and splashed ice-cold water on her face to be sure she was awake. Nora came back in the room and grabbed the piece of paper to read it again and again. *My girl is getting married. It is so fast; I do not even know him. My girl is getting married; how am I going to handle it? We have no money. I know that the boy's family has to pay for the wedding, but they have no money, either. Ok, I have to get to work and I have all the time in the world to think about it. I will talk to Ana when I get back from work. God, I am asking you again to take all these in your hands; there is not much I can do.*

Nora let Sophia sleep too, knowing that Ana would take care of her and get her ready for school. Every time she had extra time, she helped Sophia like she was her own mother.

Ana woke up, went directly to Sophia, and announced, "Sophia, wake up, wake up; I am getting married!" Ana gently shook Sophia's tiny body. "Sophia, I love you... wake up."

"Stop," she said. "You scared me. Let me sleep."

"No, wake up. I want to tell you how happy I am."

Sophia wasn't even eleven years old and she didn't care about weddings, but seeing her sister so happy was something new. "It is Alex, am I right?"

"Who else, silly? Of course, it is Alex! I love him."

"Ok. Good for you. Now let me sleep a few more minutes!"

Ana realized she was acting ridiculous and let Sophia sleep a little bit more.

When Alex called later on during the day, Ana told him how excited everybody would be about the wedding. She'd called Aunt Maria earlier in the day to share her happiness with her aunt and cousins. She had to let her brother know about it. Maybe their weddings could be close to each other, time wise.

"Alex, I'm so happy."

"Nobody could be happier than I am. The time flies by and I don't even know what I am doing."

"Me too, Alex. I am at work now, so I'll talk to you later on."

Alex had more time than Ana, even if he was studying for his finals. He admired how devoted she was to her work and to her family. He remembered the advice he received from his friends when they were getting together... do not get married young, wait. But how could he wait when he'd found such a girl? "She will be mine; I don't care. I know I am young, too young, but something tells me that we will be together forever. I know it—I feel it. It will be hard, but love will make everything possible."

* * * *

On the other side of the town, Ana's coworkers were telling her to not be in a hurry, to wait, to get to know Alex better. They shared stories about bad marriages and gave examples of different situations.

Ana let them talk, but she knew the answer—she would marry Alex. She knew he was the one—the only one.

Then a few weeks before Alex's graduation, Ana and Alex got married. Early in the morning, family and friends came to congratulate the new couple getting married at City Hall, like the law required. This was the only recognizable document of a marriage. Both of them had been advised to not get married in church, because it wasn't "healthy or politically correct" to be seen in church, any church. Alex, especially, got so many hints to stay away from church and to have only the legal ceremony, but he didn't listen to anybody. He knew this wouldn't look good, but he and his bride wanted to be married in church, to receive the Christian Orthodox blessings.

Ana loved the smell of incense, and the wedding ceremony made her feel closer to God. Both of them wanted to say, "I do" in front of God. It was so powerful, and represented a firm commitment to each other. No advice could make them give up the church ceremony. Ana wished they could have married in her church, the one across from her childhood home, but that had been demolished by the new regime to make room for more villas. Ana's school had been demolished and many houses disappeared for the same purpose.

Alex and Ana choose a beautiful church that was still standing and fully covered with painted icons. It had a special feeling, peaceful and solemn. The wedding was nicer than they thought it would be. Barely having enough money for any wedding, Ana certainly hadn't expected it to be such a nice wedding, with people coming from everywhere to congratulate the new couple. It seemed like all their family members contributed to their happiness. Even though Alex had to borrow some money to buy wedding bands for his bride and himself. He had them engraved with their names and the wedding date. No diamonds, no honeymoon.

Only love and it was everywhere! Friends and family were giving the newly married couple gifts and money. And people enjoyed the modest wedding so much, it felt like it was everybody's wedding. The food was delicious, made with love, and guests had fun dancing all night long.

Before the wedding, Alex had asked Ana if she would agree to live with his family during his six months of service in the army. Ana couldn't be happier. Any place would be much better than living under the same roof with her stepfather.

"Of course, I would love to live there, waiting for you," she agreed. "I will get to know them better than I know you!"

"My mom will be so happy; she was afraid you would say no because our house is not big enough."

"It's not the home, it's the people. Your family will be mine and small or big, it's the love that counts."

Alex found himself thanking God for sending such a soul in his way. "Ana, I know my family will adore you. My two sisters are busy working all day long; they are very good sisters. And my parents will be there for you. I am glad you said yes."

Right after the wedding, Ana moved in with Alex's parents. His sisters lived on the other side of the house, next to their aunt. Ana went back to work right after the wedding weekend, and Alex was ready for his exams. He had to study hard; he wanted to graduate with honor. The first day of army service was coming fast and the thought of leaving his wife for six months bothered him.

* * * *

"Mom, I miss Ana so much! Let's go and see her, please," Sophia asked Nora.

"She was here two days ago, you saw her."

"I know, but I am so used to doing my homework with her, talking to her, playing with her."

"Ok, we can go. Let me find some time and I promise, we'll go there."

When Nora and Sophia finally arrived at Ana's new home, they saw a long table under the grapevine with Ana and her in-laws having a good time. Nora hadn't seen her daughter so happy since she told her about her love for Alex. Thanking God for what she saw, Titus's image came to her mind. She missed her first husband, Ana and Bob's father.

Then, she thought of Nick, and how differently he treated her children from his own child. A blind person could have seen the difference. His attention, his presents, everything he had, it was only for Sophia! This man never realized that Ana and Bob could be hurt by his behavior. Her children weren't looking for presents or gifts; the only thing they wanted was a father's love.

She knew her daughter could have lived with them until Alex finished his service duty, but she preferred to live with his family. And Nora knew the reason—Ana's stepfather. With that thought,

Nora tried to be present with her mind and her heart now that she was here with Ana and her new family.

Sophia ran toward Ana and hugged her with all the strength in her tiny body. "Why did you leave me? Why? I miss you. The apartment is empty without you."

"I didn't run from you. I got married. I am a married woman now and things have changed. I have a new family now."

"What does that mean, a new family? What about us?"

"You will always be my family, my blood family, and I love you. I wish I lived closer, so we could do your homework together."

"Mom misses you too! Now she sleeps in my bed."

Ana knew her mom wasn't happy and she would like to help her, but there was nothing she could do.

Sophia and Nora had an unbelievably good time there; Alex's family had something special. They were so genuine, so pure, making everybody welcome and wishing they would come back soon. They shared things and had a nice family talk—the kind of talks that brought people closer.

Ana felt extremely happy to see them together, like a good family.

Nora was satisfied to see how her daughter's in-laws were taking care of her, treating her like their own daughter. The difference stroked her thoughts again. *Why couldn't Nick be like these people? Why didn't he see what a good daughter we had? Why is he so cold? This man is an iceberg. I wish I had never married him.* The time came to say goodbye and go home.

"Sophia, let's go home; it's getting late."

"No, I want to stay here. I like it here. I want to move here."

They all laughed hearing what Sophia said. Finally, they left and went home. When they arrived at their apartment, as soon as they opened the door, Sophia had a weird feeling, unusual for an eleven-year-old child. She compared their apartment with the place where her sister lived. "Something is missing here! Mom, I like it there more, where Ana lives," she said, looking around the apartment like it was the first time she noticed the place.

Nora couldn't take a step; she was shocked by what Sophia said.

Even Sophia feels this way? She is so young. Is it so obvious? She is right. Something is missing here, and I know what it is. Love!"

Nora tried to change the subject of the conversation, to not let Sophia see what she felt. Their apartment was an ice cave and not because of the temperature.

She realized finally that one single person could destroy everything.

* * * *

Six months had sailed by, and Ana felt like she'd lived here forever.

"Alex is coming home next week, next week, next week," Ana announced. She opened all the doors so everybody could hear. "Let's get ready!"

"How?" Alex's mother asked. "What should we do?"

"I don't know, but we have to do something. He's coming home."

"I will cook his special food that he likes so much, or better, let you cook for him," she said with a smile.

"Are you sure I can cook like you? No, for sure, but I want to try. I've watched you cook, and let's hope I picked up a thing or two."

Mother and daughter-in-law started planning step by step, preparing for Alex's day, when he would finally be reunited with his wife and his family.

Everybody got involved.

When Alex arrived, he couldn't believe how the yard looked. He felt their love in everything and it showed in each detail. Ana looked absolutely radiant and she had eyes only for her husband. Alex hugged her so much that she couldn't move. "Ana, it is impossible to tell you how much I missed you. I cannot say in words what was in my heart and in my mind during these long six months. I am such a lucky guy that somebody waited so long for me. And that the person waiting happens to be the love of my life, my wife."

"I feel the same way, but let's have dinner and celebrate the event."

"Ana, now we can say that we are married! Tomorrow, we are going to start a new life, as a married couple."

"I know. I counted all the minutes, all the days, waiting for this day to come. Now we are husband and wife. We are so blessed to have so much love, from each other and for absolutely everybody around us, family and friends. Alex, we don't need a honeymoon to be happy."

"Ana, and Mom, can you come here? I have good news."

Stephanie came in a hurry, curious to find out what her son had to say. She wished Alex's father could be here. He worked in a small town, two hours away from home, and came home only on the weekends. It often made Stephanie feel like she was a mother and a father at the same time.

"I received an offer to work at the former king's palace. Now the place is called the palace of the pioneers. They want me to teach sports to children, teenagers, like swimming, tennis, and sport shooting, and to educate them. You all know how much I love children," Alex said, looking deep in Ana's eyes. "Am I lucky or what? If you could see how that place looks, you wouldn't believe I will be working there. Can you imagine me working in the same place where our king lived?"

"Alex, stop, please. You are saying too many things, too fast. Take your time and explain to us… who is 'they'?"

"*They* means the government, the Party."

"Do you mean the Communist Party?"

"Yes, you know you can be dead without being a member of their party."

"I know," Ana said, looking sad, but excited for her husband to get a good job.

"Ana, I love children. I hope to be in charge of at least ten children and teach them all I know."

Stephanie and Ana looked at each other and had a good laugh.

She couldn't be happier than to see her son becoming a real man. Her heart was glad and beating fast. She looked at them and she thanked God for giving the best wife to her son. She let them talk and went into the kitchen to get dinner ready. Ana soon returned and helped her finish preparing the food and setting up the table.

* * * *

Ana's job gave her many rewards and she felt appreciated there. She hadn't forgotten about college; it was always somewhere in her mind.

Alex came home from work and asked Ana if she could join him at a winter camp in the mountains. He had to go there with a large group of children and teach them how to ski. She wasn't sure she could get the time off, but she tried. Her boss was so pleased with Ana's work that he agreed and gave her time off to be with her husband.

Alex and Ana went to the mountains, surrounded by the whole group of children. It felt like the honeymoon they never had. Ana tried to ski, but she was afraid of falling. She couldn't believe she could have so much fun, even when she wasn't skiing.

Coming inside the cabin, the fireplace, the hot cider, and the hot tea worked together warming up their bodies and making them feel relaxed and happy.

"Ana, thank you for coming with me. I am so happy."

"I am happier than I can say. I wish I could come more often, but my job is so much different than yours."

They had the time of their new, young, married life. Ana promised herself she would try to get time off more often, so they could spend time together.

* * * *

Ana discovered a book to help her learn English by herself, without a teacher. She felt scared at first, seeing how thick the book was, but day by day, she was getting better and loved each word she learned. Her brain was like a sponge, absorbing everything.

One day, she told her mom, "Mom, I feel like this language has a meaning for me! It soothes my mind and my heart. I love this language. I wish I knew somebody who speaks it.

"I don't feel the same with my French. Do you remember how many years I studied French? I like the French language, but this language, I love it. It is so sweet, so different. It is kind of hard to twist your tongue and to pronounce the letter 'R' softer, but practice will make it perfect. Keep learning, Ana; who knows? One day, you are going to need it."

What a premonition her mom had!

After summer arrived, Ana and Alex took a short but nice vacation at the shore of the Black Sea. What a beautiful place it was too. Alex's job gave him access to some fancy hotels where foreigners were staying. They became friends with two couples from West Germany. Young, gorgeous people and so sweet, that wanted to spend their vacation on the Black Sea's shore. It wasn't only amazingly beautiful, but also inexpensive for people from other countries.

Alex and Ana were afraid to be seen with foreigners, especially from a western country. They could lose their jobs, but the time they spent together was so wonderful, it made them forget about reality.

Their conversations were mostly about Romania, how pretty it was.

"You have everything in this country," one of their German friends said. "Huge mountains, the Danube, the Black Sea, castles, monasteries, history, so much history! Romania has castles, palaces everywhere, and above all, the people, such friendly people. Everybody smiles and you can see on their faces how sincere they are."

"I know," Ana answered, biting her tongue so she wouldn't say what was really on her mind: "Yes, the country is so beautiful, but the government is destroying everything, day by day. Romania is a very rich country, with gold, oil, and natural treasures, but the Russians take most of these to their country. We live under the Russian boot. We have to learn the Russian language in school and it isn't optional." Ana didn't want her friends to feel sorry for them. She and Alex were very proud of their country; it was the place where they were born and they loved it.

One of the couples came from a big city and they had a nice income, without graduating college. Ana couldn't believe somebody could have so much money without going to college. She was taught that you couldn't do anything without college.

They decided to have dinner at a nice terrace on the shore. The weather was perfect and the breeze was spreading salty air from the sea. It was heaven; Alex had his arms around Ana's shoulders, holding her close to his body. He didn't want this moment to end.

When they arrived at the restaurant, their German friends were already there.

Ana and Alex looked at each other and admired the famous German punctuality.

They had a good time, even though Ana's English wasn't as good as she wanted it to be; the sign language worked wonders. Ana's words made their friendship stronger.

But where there was love, there was a way. They became good friends, and when that couple went back to Germany, Ana and Alex started receiving packages with clothes, toiletries, shoes, and other presents. It wasn't a good thing for the new couple to have a relationship with "capitalist" couples and receive goods from them, but Ana and Alex were young and dreaming for a better life. Their vacation was coming to an end.

Ana recalled her mom saying, "Keep learning English; who knows? One day, you might need it."

Mothers always know. Just as Nora had known when Ana was a beautiful young woman that she would become beautiful and elegant. She thought the gifts from the German couple were beautiful and elegant. Ana hadn't owned that kind of clothing since her father was alive! A long, long time ago.

* * * *

It had been a busy week at work and Ana had a deadline on her project, so she was coming in earlier in the morning and going home later in the evening. She thought her coworkers were busy with their own work and they were concentrating on finishing the project also.

But there was a person that couldn't do anything else but think of Ana. Everybody feared Stan because he was one of the leaders of the Communist organization where Ana worked. He was an engineer, married, but it seemed he liked women and tried to intimidate them with his political power.

One day, he approached Ana and said, with a professional tone, "Ana, next week, we have to go to a job site to test some of the prototypes we made, and I put you on the list."

"Ok, sir, I will do what I have to do."

It was getting dark outside, and Ana put her drawing tools in the drawer, grabbed her purse, and tried to open the door.

Suddenly, he closed the door and put his arm around Ana's shoulders. Stan said, "Ana, I love you. We are alone; don't be scared."

Ana stepped back and said, "Sir, please, take your hands off me and let me leave."

"I will let you leave, but if you say something about this, nobody will believe you and you will lose your job."

Ana left the office furious, so angry that she couldn't even cry. Ana decided not to say anything to Alex; she knew her husband wouldn't let her go back to work. But she needed to talk to her cousin Peter and tell him what just happened. She arrived home and Alex was waiting for her, all smiles and love.

"Are you ok? You look so sad!"

"Do I? No, I am only tired. Let's have dinner."

The next day, Ana talked to her cousin about the incident. Peter couldn't believe what he heard and was determined to have a serious talk with his colleague. He had a moral responsibility for his cousin; he considered Ana his sister and he promised he would take care of her when her father passed away. He knew Ana was married, but like Ana, he didn't want Alex to be involved in this. Peter knew he could lose his job, because that engineer had a higher political position, but he had to protect Ana.

Stan could become his enemy, and put his job in jeopardy. The Communists ruled the country, and you couldn't play games with the Communist Party. It was a dangerous situation, but family was stronger than everything, so he approached his colleague and asked him to go for a walk around the building.

Peter said, "If you ever touch my cousin or even dare to say something to her, I will inform our superiors and most importantly, your wife, your family. Hope I am clear enough. We have to be professional; we have to collaborate and be on good terms. I will not say one word to anybody. So, take care of your behavior and nobody will ever know about what you did, but I've warned you."

Since that day, nobody bothered Ana. Everything went back to normal. Ana kept doing her job—a really good job.

* * * *

Two years passed by, full of love and living as a young, happy married couple.

Ana and Alex put a down payment on a small apartment and they moved in as soon as the building was ready. Both of them missed the time spent with Alex's family, so almost every evening they went there to chat and hug their loved ones.

One day, Ana came home with a big smile on her face. Alex was so happy to see her that way. He asked her, "Did you get another promotion?"

"No, but I have been promoted to become a mother!"

"What? You're pregnant? Thank you, God! I will be a father!"

"I'm happy too, but I already started worrying about how hard it will be to raise a child these days. I see people around me, and I see how much they struggle to do the right things for their kids. It won't be easy, I know, and that's why I let almost three years pass since we got married, to be sure we could do it. But I realized things aren't getting any better, so we will do what everybody does."

"How can you talk like this? We're going to have a child, that's all that matters. Our child! Let's go to everybody's homes, all our relatives, and tell them the good news. Right now, let's go."

"My God, you are crazy! Ok, let's go; you're contagious in your craziness. I'm trying to think logically, but you're right. We're going to have a baby, our baby. Let's go."

She loved her husband's enthusiasm, and it reminded her of how he wanted to have ten children! Ana knew how blessed she was to have such a good man in her life, on her side.

Soon, everybody knew about their happy news. Bob already had a one-year-old son. Peter also had a one-year-old son; the family was getting larger. And what a family they had—loving and helping each other.

CHAPTER ELEVEN

Ana's pregnancy didn't slow her down; she never missed a work day. She was all smiles and she had a glow of happiness. Being young and healthy, she expected her pregnancy to go smoothly with no problems. When she was just beyond six months pregnant, something happened that she wasn't prepared for. She looked at one of her female coworkers and asked her to come closer to her.

"Are you ok? You look like you saw a ghost."

"I think my water broke. Please call the ambulance and my husband; this is his phone number," Ana said, holding her stomach. "I am so scared. I don't know what to do."

The ambulance took her to the closest hospital.

When Alex found out about what happened, he called Maria right away. Not only was Maria a midwife, but she was like a mother to Ana. Maria went to the hospital and tried to find Ana's doctor, a good friend of hers, Dr. Isad. This doctor had been taking care of Ana from the beginning of her pregnancy.

When she heard about Ana's incident, she knew the complications would be hard to deal with. Maria called Dr. Isad and explained to him the situation, asking him to hurry up and come to the hospital as soon as he could.

The doctor had been playing poker with his friends, so he wasn't too happy to leave the game. He complained about this as soon as he arrived at the hospital.

Ana was in excruciating pain, but she tried to be as quiet as she could. The nurse tried to explain to her that a miscarriage has occurred and that the baby couldn't and wouldn't survive.

Ana kept saying, "I want my baby; I want my baby."

"Ana, you cannot have this baby; it is a miscarriage. The baby cannot survive without the fluid you had, and now that liquid is gone. You have to understand; it is impossible. You and your husband are young, and you can have another baby after this."

"No, I want my baby! Help me, please," Ana desperately implored the doctor and the nurses.

"What's happened?" Dr. Isad asked Ana. "Did you lift something heavy?"

"No, I was in my office and suddenly, water started running down my legs."

"Ana, I have to apply forceps to pull the baby out."

Ana was in such pain that she hadn't even heard what the doctor said. He pulled the baby's head with the forceps carelessly, being in a hurry to return to his poker game. He was finishing what he was doing when he got interrupted by a phone call. He didn't care about the baby or the mother! His addiction was stronger than his obligations as a doctor. Dr. Isad gave the baby to his nurse and told her to leave it on the tray, on the floor. He considered the baby a miscarriage and felt sure that she, because it was a baby girl, wouldn't survive.

The nurse was skeptical, but she had to do what the doctor told her to do. She put the baby girl in the tray and the tray on the floor. Maria wasn't allowed to be in the operating room. Otherwise, this would have never happened. Ana had no more voice to cry or scream for her baby; she was exhausted.

When she did speak, her voice was only a whisper, "I want my baby; please, help me."

Dr. Isad finished cleaning up, so he could leave when he realized the baby girl was still breathing; he couldn't believe how strong that baby was. He told the nurse to grab the baby and put her in an incubator. He thought she would probably die there. She was a premature baby, stage three, and it was impossible to survive, according to his knowledge. The baby's face was black and blue from the broken vessels in her brain. The left half of her face was completely black from the chin all the way to the hair line and beyond. The forceps had been incorrectly applied and destroyed valuable cells in the baby's brain, and he knew it; he knew exactly what he did! "At least, Ana cannot say that I didn't try to save her child."

Precious minutes were lost, precious seconds were wasted on the tray, on the floor.

Dr. Isad returned to his poker game, getting absorbed by his passion for gambling and completely forgetting about what he just did, changing somebody's life forever, a whole family's fate.

* * * *

Alex rushed to the hospital, but he wasn't allowed to be anywhere close to the maternity hallway. The rules were very strict. He asked Maria to not forget about him and to come and talk to him so he would know about his wife and what happened with the baby. Maria promised to come as soon as she could find out something about Ana and the baby. Alex walked up and down an empty hallway trying to figure out how his wife was doing and afraid to think of his child, knowing the term of the pregnancy.

Maria went inside the pavilion and what she saw shook her body; being a midwife for years and years, the image she just witnessed was worse than any other image she'd ever seen before. The small, tiny body in the incubator with a face half-bruised! My God, what had this doctor done? She almost fainted.

The nurse helped her to sit down and she tried to justify her actions. "The doctor told me to put the baby on a tray and to put the tray on the floor," she said, crying. "I had to do it. I am so sorry. He said that the baby was a miscarriage and wouldn't survive."

"It is not your fault," Maria said, "You did what he told you to do. Is the baby a girl or a boy?"

"A girl," she said through her tears.

Maria knew how much Ana wanted to have a girl. She loved Sophia so much, she wanted another Sophia.

"Is my niece ok? I have to see her."

The nurse took Maria to Ana's bed. It was a large room, and

ugly, lined with many beds. Maria was amazed how good her niece looked after such a hard labor and such a difficult delivery. Thinking about the little girl's face, Maria considered that Dr. Isad had been in a hurry, not letting the forceps go in, but forcing them in. Her anger boiled beneath the surface. "You look so good, Ana! Congratulations, you have a baby girl, and soon, you will hold her in your arms."

Ana thanked her aunt, but she noticed right away that Maria hadn't said, *"A healthy, beautiful baby girl,"* she only said, *"A baby girl."* "I am so glad she's alive! I have to see her."

"You will, but you have to wait a little while. Alex is outside and he asked me to give you a hug."

"He wants to see his baby too. I know."

"Don't worry, he will. Now get some rest. I will stay here with you all day."

* * * *

Ana couldn't sleep. She had to see her baby. The nurse promised to take her to the incubator, so she could meet her newborn baby girl.

Alex and Ana hadn't decided what name to give to their baby. Six days went by, and Ana still hadn't seen her daughter.

"There must be something really wrong if they won't let me hold her," she told Maria. "Please, tell me what is going on. It drives me insane to know I am so close to my baby and I can't hold her in my arms."

"Didn't I promise you that I would keep you informed with everything, and that when the time comes, you will see your baby girl?"

"Yes, but I cannot take it anymore."

Maria was there with her niece, every day. She was keeping her informed about how the baby was doing.

The doctor finished his routine visits and Ana's bed was the last patient.

You could see on his face that he had no remorse for what he did to Ana's baby. His face was all smiles, like nothing happened. "Ana, your baby is doing great, but she has to be in the incubator for at least one more month, till she gains the necessary weight, so you can take her home. The incubator replaces your womb, so she stays warm and we feed her. If you want to go home, you can, and then you can come back and visit her."

"I want to see her now, right now."

"Ok, I will tell the nurse to take care of this. Tell your husband to go to City Hall and register the baby. Now, I am positive she will survive. Give her a name, and then tell him to bring back the birth certificate so we can have a copy of it. This way we can put her name on the incubator."

"I will. I am not going home. I will stay here with her, till we go home together, mother and daughter. I am not leaving the hospital."

"Ok, but there is not much you can do here; you will be bored."

Ana went to see her baby for the first time. "Oh my God, she is so small! Is that what three pounds looks like? Alex will be shocked! I will ask all the nursing mothers to give me some of their milk so my baby will have breast milk. It is the best thing I can do for her right at this moment. The milk from those mothers would be a precious gift for my baby."

Ana went back in her hospital room and cried until her eyes were dry. "I will love and take care of this child with all my heart. I hope and pray to God that she will be ok. What a trauma to start your life like this!"

When Alex was allowed to see his baby for the first time, he was so shocked that he ran down the stairs, crying. It was an instinct reaction. He couldn't control his reaction; he was completely stunned. He realized he was the father of that tiny baby and would love her forever.

Ana understood why her husband ran from the window. She had the same feeling when she saw her daughter for the first time, but she stayed glued to the window! The nurse explained to her that nobody was allowed inside but the nurses and doctors.

Ana realized it would be a very long time before she could leave the hospital with her newborn baby, so she started visiting all the patients, offering help to the mothers that just had their babies, helping them to walk, go to the bathroom, hold their babies, change the sheets, everything that was needed.

Ana's baby was getting breast milk from all the mothers in that hospital, the best gift she could get to grow and be healthy.

* * * *

"Sarah! Sarah!" Ana repeated the name Alex had chosen for their child.

Alex asked Ana what name she wanted, but she let him be the one to name her. What a beautiful, strong name; she loved her new daughter's name. Alex brought back the baby's birth certificate, so now their baby was officially registered.

He arrived every single day to see Ana and the baby in the hospital.

"Can you believe how much she has grown?" Ana said to him. "She gets milk from all the mothers here. They adopted her and everybody is happy to give her breast milk."

"I miss you, and the apartment is so empty without you."

"Don't worry; soon it will be very loud. She will cry and keep us up."

"You didn't say I miss you too," Alex noticed.

"I do miss you, but my mind is only full of our baby."

* * * *

Two months went by, two months without Ana, being alone in his apartment. Alex's family was concerned and everybody tried to help him to not feel lonely. They went to the hospital to see how Ana and the baby were doing.

The doctor came in the room and said, "Ok, you can go home with your baby today. She has gained enough weight and she is doing very well."

They were excited. They could go home, finally.

A nurse came and instructed them where to take the baby for

immunizations and check-ups. She gave Ana a prescription for special milk that Sarah had to drink and wished them good luck. The nurse prayed on her way out that the baby would be ok.

Alex prepared everything for Ana and the baby, being so happy to take them home. Sarah ate normally and looked like any other baby her age.

Their German friends knew about the whole situation and sent packages including special children's vitamins that nobody she knew had heard about. Ana took those vitamins and the special milk she received from her friends and showed it to the baby's pediatrician. He checked the labels and was excited that Ana would be able to give these to her baby. And he was right; Sarah looked like a baby doll. She was beautiful and had a happy face; the bruise from her left side was almost gone. Sarah was growing just like a weed, making everybody happy and feel at ease playing with her.

Ana went back to work every day, except Sundays. That day she had to do everything for her family, especially cooking and food shopping—whatever food she could find.

Alex was happy to play with Sarah. Everybody could see the bond between father and daughter; they were so happy together. One afternoon, Alex and Ana went for a walk in the park with Sarah in the stroller.

"I went to see her pediatrician today," Ana said.

"And what did he say? Is everything ok? She looks amazing, doesn't she?"

"I asked him why Sarah cannot sit without being propped between pillows and he advised us to be patient. He said it would take her more time to do what other children do because she was a premature baby, stage three. I told him how Sarah is trying to get up on her knees, but she cannot stay there. Maybe he is right? We just have to wait."

"Don't worry," Alex said. "Our baby will be ok, I adore her."

Nora alternated taking care of Sarah with Alex's mother Stephanie. What a good woman she was. Ana considered herself very lucky to have such a good mother-in-law; it was like having two mothers. Sarah was surrounded by love and care, from everybody and from everywhere.

Ana wasn't the only one having the time of her life. Sophia was in love with her high school sweetheart, Arthur, who was two years older than her and crazy about her. They both enjoyed playing with Sarah, holding her and making her laugh. Ana used that time to do things around the apartment, getting ready for work, cooking, making appointments, washing clothes by hand, and working hard. Ana felt grateful to get help, and Sarah was grateful to spend time with Sophia and her boyfriend.

Ana and Alex were showered in love from their neighbors, too. "Alex, you are the best father," they told him all the time. "Every time we see you, you're taking care of your baby. Sarah is a lucky child."

Alex's heart was full of hope and dreams. He could see himself teaching Sarah how to swim, play tennis, and even skiing, possibly to make her a champion.

"Tomorrow, the nurse is coming," Ana told her husband. "She's a nice lady and she makes Sarah laugh."

"Good, you should be nice too. Give me a hug, please."

The nurse came on time, and Ana felt glad because she wouldn't be late for work. Even though Ana loved what she was doing at her job, since she'd had the baby, she wanted to stay home with her all the time, but they couldn't afford such a luxury.

Sarah smiled when she saw the nurse. She was now ten months old.

"Ana, could you take Sarah for an MRI to be sure everything is ok?" she said when she finished her exam.

"Why? What do you think? Is something wrong with her? Tell me, please."

"I don't know what to say. I see quite a few babies a day, and I think, by now, Sarah should sit and stand—with help, of course. I know she was born premature, but because of how the doctor used the forceps to get her out, I would suggest having this test done."

"Thank you for telling me. I will take her for the test."

Alex came home that night and found Ana in tears. "What's happened? Why are you crying? Where is Sarah?"

"She's sleeping. The nurse thinks there's something wrong with her."

"No, there is nothing wrong with her. She's just behind the other babies her age because she was a preemie, and she's taking longer to be like the other babies."

"I know, but we have to have this test done."

Ana and Alex took time off to go together for the test. Sarah was happy and smiling. They went to the best neurological institute with the best doctors. They wanted absolutely the best for their daughter. The test was painless but hard to perform because the baby had to be completely still.

The test result was brutal: cerebral palsy. The forceps and how they were used by the doctor, destroyed parts of the movement center of Sarah's brain, explaining the bruised face. She had a black spot in her brain, dead nerve cells, dead cells.

Suddenly the future, Sarah's and for all the family members who adored her seemed to now be covered by thick, dark gray clouds. There are things in life that cannot be explained or understood, why they happened.

Ana and Alex refused to let the black stamp mark their lives. They had a moral obligation for their baby.

* * * *

"Alex, Sarah's birthday is coming soon; we better get prepared. Everybody will come to our apartment to celebrate her first birthday."

The family got together with flowers, balloons, cake, and music to make their place a happy place again.

The next day, they took Sarah for a walk in the park in the stroller. They started looking at the other babies that were close to Sarah's age and noticed the differences; the way they sat, stood, crawled, twisted, moved, everything. Now they were able to see what other people could see looking at their daughter.

"I started doing exercises with Sarah, and she enjoyed it; she cooperated."

"What do you mean? Cooperated?"

"When I pushed her leg, she pushed back towards me. I think this is a good sign."

"Of course," Alex said. "She'll be ok. We are going to do everything the doctor tells us to do."

"Just to hear the word 'doctor' makes me sick. Why did he have to use that horrible instrument? The baby was so small, and—do you know what?—I don't think it was the instrument, but it was the way he used it."

"I know it. He should be in jail."

"I made an appointment with a neurosurgeon. I can't wait to see what his opinion is."

"Let's go back home, give Sarah a good bath and a nice massage. She already likes the good stuff. Look at her, how beautiful she is. She is my precious baby girl, and I love both of you so much. I live for you."

* * * *

"What did the doctor say?" Nora asked her daughter.

"Alex and I are going tomorrow to see the doctor. Mom, tell me, why did this have to happen to my child, to us, to all of us? What did I do wrong? I've never even killed a fly! I have never hurt anybody, not even with words. Why? Why? Mom, I am devastated. My baby isn't right! That doctor destroyed her and us, destroyed her life, her future. Why?"

"We don't choose our destiny; it is given to us, and we just obey it."

"How can I obey when my child suffers, when I see my own child facing a tougher world as a paralyzed woman?"

"Stop talking like this; miracles happen all the time. Pray that she will be able to walk, to have a normal life. She's already smart, talking a lot more than other babies her age. It is a pleasure for me to take care of her. I'm so impressed with how many words she knows and how much she talks. I wish I were retired, so I could be with her all the time. Tomorrow, I'll bring Sophia to play with Sarah.

I know she and Arthur send their love."

"I miss my sister so much, Mom. Every time she comes, I have to use the time she plays with Sarah to do other things that I don't have time for. I'm so glad she has a boyfriend. I like him. Now my time is so divided, Sarah and work, Sarah and doctors."

"What about Alex? Do you make time for him?"

"No, not like before! He knows how hard it is to take care of all the things that pile on in our lives. At least, where he works, he is surrounded by normal, happy children and all his coworkers are healthy and fit. It's their job to look good and to keep in good shape. He tried to refuse some of the summer camps where he has been directed to go and we are waiting for his boss answer. I know it will be hard without him, but if he has to go, it is his job and he has to go. Thank God, I have you and Stephanie."

Nora tried to get her daughter to understand that Alex worked in a different environment, a lot different than he had at home. The young teachers that he worked with were beautiful and most of them there were single. She knew about them from talking with Alex. He was so sincere that he told his family everything going on at work. Beauty, health, fitness, normality, everything at work brought him joy simply by being there.

Ana seemed too preoccupied with her child's development to pay attention to all the details, but Nora was all ears. Her life experience had made her aware and she tried to show Ana that she needed to take care of her husband, to not neglect him.

Coming home, everything for Alex changed into suffering, pain, and uncertainty.

To see your own child not being able to walk, or being able to enjoy what all the kids around her were enjoying. Love was the only thing that was making him strong enough to resist all the temptations and comparisons he was making while looking around him.

* * * *

The doctor's office was elegant but cold. It felt like nothing good could come out of it. And this was the truth, unfortunately. The doctor "played" with Sarah, testing her motor and intellectual abilities.

"Ana," he said, "Sarah has a typical case of cerebral palsy. Her brain, her intellect will be in a 'normal range' and 'normal' is a very wide field. She will talk—she already talks more than other kids, but her motor skills are compromised."

"So, what can be done?" Alex asked the doctor with sadness in his voice.

"She will need physical therapy and lots of surgeries. It will take a couple of years to get some results."

"What do you mean a couple of years? She won't be able to walk?"

"Maybe with a walker, but for now we have to lessen her spasticity, in other words, she has to have surgeries to elongate her tendons."

When the appointment was over, Ana and Alex looked like two devastated people, with their shoulders down, no hope in their hearts, their dreams killed. The sky fell on their minds and bodies. They looked at each other with tears in their eyes.

"Alex, I don't want Sarah to suffer. I'm not going to let them cut her. We have to see another doctor. I'll make an appointment and go and get a second opinion."

"You're right. We have to see what another doctor says."

Ana made the appointment and the doctor confirmed the diagnosis! It was absolutely the same, the same sentence. It was the sentence for Sarah's life. On the way home, not even one word was said. Sarah smiled trying to get their attention. Seeing her smiling made their feelings heavier, and guilty.

"We will be ok. God loves us. We didn't do anything wrong. Ana, we will be ok. I love you both so much."

She gave Alex no answer, and he thought maybe she hadn't heard his words. The devastation covered Ana and it dug deep into her soul.

Sarah had to undergo multiple surgeries and physical therapy sessions for over a two- year period. She had so much pain and tears, but she was still smiling. What an amazing child! Ana and Alex cried more than their child did. The love Sarah had from everybody was a beautiful gift.

One day, early in the morning, somebody knocked at their apartment door. Ana, holding Sarah in her arms, opened the door and saw two women standing there. Both women looked like government employees, holding a suitcase and folders.

"Are you Ana Volk?"

"Yes, I am. Who are you?"

"We represent the department of families with children and we want you to sign this document. Our department is considering taking away your child and putting her in a special institution, so you can be dedicated to your work and to our party."

Normally, Ana would invite those women to come inside, offer them some tea or coffee, but when she heard their reason for visiting, she almost fainted. Thank God, she didn't drop Sarah on the floor. Holding her child tight, Ana took a step forward and, with a very calm and firm voice, she said, "If somebody else dares to knock at my door again, asking for my child, to take away my child, I will kill that person, and if you don't disappear right now, I will kill you too. You have my word."

The two women ran as fast as they could. Ana went back inside the apartment, holding her daughter close to her chest. She tried to keep the tears from pouring down her face, but she couldn't stop them. And Sarah, the poor child, she had no idea what just happened but she started crying too, seeing her mama crying.

Ana covered her baby in kisses and said, "Nobody will ever take you away from me! I will give my life for you. I love you, baby; I will sacrifice everything I have to see you better, to have a better life. Your father and I adore you."

Alex came home, full of love and all smiles, but seeing his wife's face, he stopped right in the hallway. "Are you ok? Is something wrong with Sarah? Where is she?"

"Sarah is ok. She is taking a nap now. How are you? How was your day?"

"Oh no, tell me about you, why did you cry? What's happened?"

"Alex, let's eat first, then we'll sit down and I'll tell you what this is all about. Everything will be just fine."

"No, I cannot eat and see your face like this. Something terrible must have happened. If Sarah is ok, something must have happened at work. Did they fire you?"

"Not yet, but with the many 'sick days' I took for Sarah's surgeries, it wouldn't shock me to find out that I could lose my job. But I cannot believe how wonderful my coworkers are. They cover for me; they work on my part of the project without being paid extra money. They know that I would do the same thing for them. What a group of people! This regime is awful, but the people are amazing. I feel sorry for all of us."

"I know we are blessed in so many ways. How was your day?"

"No, tell me about yours," Ana said, trying to postpone the real subject.

"Oh, today, I started working with a nine-year-old boy. He is a genius young man. I have such a good feeling about him. I'll train him really well."

"I know you will, and he will become an Olympic champion if you train him."

"His parents invited us for dinner. They just met me and they already invited us to go to their apartment and have dinner together."

"What did you say? Did you accept the invitation?"

"I said I would talk to you first, because it is so hard for us to go out with Sarah."

"I think we should accept the invitation. We have changed so much. Before we had Sarah, we were going from one relative to another having fun, but now, everything we do is pain, tears and more pain. Sarah is our priority, and look at her, she's dreaming now; she is smiling in her sleep. Look at that smile."

"I cannot wait to come home and play with her. Ok, I can eat now, but I want to 'eat' you first. I love you."

"It feels good to hear it. It feels like a Band-Aid on my heart." They sat down, had dinner, and talked about ordinary things.

Not long after, Ana said, "Alex, somebody came today, from the government, and asked us to give up our child."

"Wait a minute, what did you say?"

Ana explained the incident and she could see Alex's eyes getting wider and angrier. "Tell me this isn't true! I think it is because no one could come up with such a morbid joke. What did you do? Don't open the door if they come back."

"I assure you they will never come back. They will have to kill me first in order to take my child away from me."

"I know this. I would do the same thing. Thank God, I wasn't home or they would have put me in jail."

* * * *

When Nora found out about the horrible thing the regime did, all she remembered were the atrocities she'd faced, including the death of her first husband, Titus. This is what the Communist Party does, but people had to live with this, under their rules. The Party dictated how people lived, what they eat, when they eat, what to see on television, where they could travel, if they were even allowed to travel.

The government was very strict about what countries people could visit because the rulers were afraid that people would open their minds by seeing how other people lived their lives and realize the degree of oppression they were under. The government decided everything for a person's destiny. Each of them were slaves of Communism without the chains, but there were heavier chains, mental ones! Nora remembered when she and Ana had to warm up food on the back of the press iron because the government decided to "cut" the gas supply to save money for the Party, so they could build monstrosities, huge ugly buildings for their rich members.

There were many times when people had to wake up in the middle of the night to cook or wash clothes, depending on the "savings schedule." Nora felt so sorry for her children, for the times they lived in. She'd had a good life when younger and everybody around her had the same, so she expected the same for her children, but—Nora couldn't stop making comparisons between the past and the present.

The war destroyed everything, and the Russians took the rest. Nora realized her job was to help Ana raise her child and be there for her when surgeries and physical therapy sessions had to be done. It was like a full-time job. Stephanie and Nora were taking turns, and they put so much love into their work. Nobody dared to come back to Ana's door to ask for the child. For sure, those women informed their superiors that they should leave that family alone because the mother was a beast. And about this she was. Don't try to touch a mother that loves her child—or try to face the women in that family.

* * * *

Ana and Alex were having dinner when he asked, "Why do we let the doctors cut Sarah so much? It's clear by now that her walking is getting worse and so obvious that it doesn't help her. So much suffering, so much pain."

"Alex, if we don't do it, if we don't agree to all these surgeries, Sarah will ask us later why we didn't do it. She would be right to ask, because who are we to decide when we aren't doctors? What if she does have a chance to walk? If we stop doing what the doctors suggest and if she never walks, then we are going to feel guilty for the rest of our lives."

"Maybe you're right; we have to do everything the doctors say." Alex realized that he had the same joy coming home to his loved ones, but something new was added to his joy—pain. A very heavy pain, a cruel and undeserved pain, to see your own child suffering and not be able to walk. Going on trips with his family, he would carry Sarah on his shoulders and play with her, pretending she was like all the other children. She was so happy, and she loved her father more than anything in the world. She was a "daddy's girl."

Ana was more than happy to see how much joy Alex was giving their child. He had a good heart and being a teacher, he knew how to approach a child, while Ana was more disciplinary.

As time went by, there were more surgeries, more pain, and Sarah started using a walker before they were ready for a wheelchair. Their apartment building had no ramp, no handrails, no wide doors, nothing for handicapped children or adults.

All the horrid buildings were the same. The government didn't want to have "physically handicapped people," and they would never do anything for them. This was one of the reasons they wanted all of these children or adults to be put in special institutions.

Sometimes the country was like a third world country. What a shame. One of the most beautiful countries in the world, that was so rich, would become a shame among European countries.

Ana's mind sometimes went back to her "desire," of going to college. Her life was so different now. Her life had changed so much with Sarah's problems. To have a handicapped child and to work six days a week, full time, didn't leave too much free time. Her fate was sealed; work and family and nothing else. She knew she was smart; she knew she could attend and graduate from a college of her choice, but going to college would take time, and all her time was dedicated to Sarah and her surgeries. It seemed that the only college she would ever be able to graduate from would be "the college of life."

She was still thirsty for knowledge, so she was reading as much as she could on her way to work and back. In the mornings, when she was taking the electrical tram or the bus, she was happy when they weren't so crowded so she could read. This was how she'd read *Gone with the Wind*, a few times, learning pages by heart.

Ana and Alex were so blessed to have a large and loving family. Their siblings had wonderful children and they were very supportive, playing with Sarah and spending time with her.

Chris and Peter were like brothers to her; the way they had grown up all together sealed their brotherhood. Bob was the only one living far away, in a different city. He wished to be closer to help his sister, but he had to be there for his soccer players and for his own family.

Life only got harder for Ana and Alex; Sarah was getting heavier and still had to be taken to her appointments, to different therapies. They decided to bring a teacher home to instruct their daughter on all the subjects children were taught in school. They made that decision because there were no schools equipped with anything to help handicapped children enter the school, use the bathrooms, or even to sit in a class.

There'd been nothing to aid her, so they had no other choice. Of course, they wanted Sarah to be in school with other children, to socialize, to feel the same as all the other kids. It would help everybody, and Sarah could be a lot happier than being alone at home with no other children around her. She had lots of love and attention, but it would be so different to be with children her age.

Sarah loved her teacher and she told her mom every day about what she learned, what color her teacher's nails were and that she was a good student. Soon, she developed a passion for poems; she loved to read poems. Reading was taking her to different worlds, meeting different people, experiencing different situations. It became a refuge.

Meanwhile, Alex's student became an Olympic medalist, bringing pride and joy to Alex because he worked so hard to train him. What an achievement! It was a much- needed celebration.

Ana felt grateful that her husband had a good job, a good position, at the university. That was only part of what still attracted her to him. Literally, she had always liked the way Alex looked, and she was definitely still in love with him, but she also knew their lives could be so different, happier, without Sarah's health problems. And there were so many, so difficult and without hope of a cure. Ana felt buried more and more by all these problems. She tried to balance her marriage life, her work and the desire to look fashionable, beautiful and put together, despite the fact that her child was handicapped.

Sometimes, she felt guilty getting dressed in a nice outfit, spraying perfume, applying makeup. She thought it was like false advertising, how what she displayed didn't represent how she felt inside her soul.

At the same time, everything she was facing gave her a sense of strength, to keep going. Nobody could guess her struggles, her pain and how she fought for a better future for her daughter. She learned how to put a "screen" between her and the world. It helped her face all the daily challenges that were coming towards her, every day.

Her child was her world and she was dedicated to Sarah's wellness.

Ana talked to God every single day; when she was done praying, she would tell herself, "I am strong; everything will be ok. I am strong. I will be even stronger. My family needs me, Alex and Sarah. I love them so much. I have been chosen to be Sarah's mother. I feel it... I know it. This is my job and it will be done very well. God knows how much I will fight for my daughter, like I already did with those two women from the government. Sarah would never be put in a special institution, to be left there to die, to starve to death, like they do to so many children."

* * * *

Alex came home from work, expecting an ordinary, loving evening with Ana and Sarah. How beautiful his girls were! He watched his wife and noticed how tired she looked, but still beautiful. Their life together was full of unpredictable, unexpected events.

If somebody examined their marriage, they would wonder how they were able to keep the flame burning, when so many "flame extinguishers" had happened. Having a child that couldn't walk and all the problems that came with this. Living in a building with stairs and no handicapped access, no ramps— living in a city they loved but that had nothing for people with physical challenges—every day was a struggle to survive, forget about being happy.

Sarah kissed her father; they played and had a good time together making Ana happy. She loved seeing Sarah happy and enjoying her time with her "papa." Sarah called her father "papa," even if everybody thought it was a name for a grandfather. She tried other names but she always came back to her "papa."

Ana helped Sarah to get ready for bed. She kissed her cheeks and said a prayer over her daughter. Alex was waiting in the kitchen so he could talk to Ana about daily things, bills, appointments, money, and a lot more. He didn't expect to hear what Ana said when she came back.

"Alex, I know you are having an affair," she said with a firm and calm voice.

In his entire life, Alex had never been so surprised. How did she find out? How could she know? Who told her? It took him a moment to get himself together, and then he answered, "No, I did not have an affair, but I tried to find a place where I can go without seeing pain around me, where everything was normal, like in so many families. Yes, I dreamed about having children that I can ski with, play tennis with, and have a parent- child relationship. I love Sarah, but every time I see her, I see pain and suffering, problems, surgeries. Ana, I'm not as strong as you are. I have to admit: I did try to find a refuge, but I couldn't do it. I know you're not going to believe me, but this is the truth."

Ana's knees "melted," her heart raced, beating hard inside her chest. "Alex, our marriage is not a prison. You can be free anytime you want, and me too. I don't need you. I have Sarah! I had numerous occasions to find a 'refuge' like you said, but you and Sarah were more important to me than anything else."

Alex tried to justify his behavior, but Ana's ears were deaf. Suddenly, she remembered how her father couldn't handle life under the Communist rules and how he took his own life, leaving her mom alone with two children. She had no right to judge her father, but the word "coward" came to her mind, much as it had come to her mother's mind, long ago. Are all men cowards? No, they aren't; at least, not all of them. Look at Bob, Chris, Cornelius—Alex's father, they had to survive and they did.

Nobody said it would be easy, but it is your duty as a Christian to do the best you could. To live for your family and for God. Life gets tough so you just have to get tougher.

Ana looked at Alex and said, "Even if you didn't have an affair, the fact that you tried to, for me, is the same thing. Tomorrow we can talk about divorce. I have to go to bed now. Good night."

The whole world was sitting heavy on Ana's shoulders, making her feel like crawling on the floor. God, it wasn't enough to have a handicapped child; now Alex? I know it is not me, or maybe, it is me? Did I neglect him? Yes, I did. Weeks in the hospital, taking care of our child, trying to do the best I could for Sarah. But how was this possible? He was with me every day, always helping, so why?

Tonight, everything had changed! Ana was suddenly angry, finding herself to still be attracted to Alex, even after she found out about what he did, but her decision was firm. She wanted to get a divorce. It was something that had never happened in her family. She would be the first one and, hopefully, the last one.

Morning came too quickly, but Ana's mind hadn't changed. She said to her husband, "Alex, I am ready to talk to you about the divorce."

He didn't say one word, kissed his daughter, and left for work.

Sarah's eyes were inquiring. She asked her mom to come closer to hug her. The moment Ana felt Sarah's arms around her, and the love coming from those arms, Ana's tears were unstoppable.

Without saying a word, Sarah kept touching her mom's hair and she kissed Ana's hands.

"Sarah, I know how much you love your father. I love him too, but he has to move out because of his job. You will still see him, but not like now."

"Do you mean my papa? No, no, I want my papa here, all the time! No, we'll move with him."

"Ok, Sarah, we'll see. Now let's get ready for your appointment."

"I don't want more surgeries Mom. It hurts so much, even the exercises hurt. Can we stop getting these, please? I've had enough."

They went to their appointment and Sarah was prescribed new foot braces to keep her knees straight.

"Mom, I would like to read more poems by Eminescu. Can you please grab the book for me?" Sarah said as soon as she came home with her mother. Eminescu was a famous poet and Sarah was in love with his poems.

"Of course, just give me few seconds to put my purse away, and I will give it to you." Ana handed the book to Sarah and she started reading her poems.

"Mom, it seems like he put a spoon of honey in each word. I want to spend my entire day reading those verses."

Ana couldn't believe what her daughter said. *I would never be able to make such a comment. What an imagination.*

Ana went and sat close to Sarah, listening to her reading. The more she listened, the more she agreed with her daughter. Ana had studied those poems in school, she loved them, but she never imagined things the way Sarah did.

It had been a new imaginary world opened for Ana to love and escape into. What a gift Sarah gave her mother; what a joy. Reading, she lived each character, every feeling, pain or happiness, love or sorrow. She always loved to read but poems weren't her thing. Until now, when Sarah opened her eyes to a different spiritual beauty.

CHAPTER TWELVE

Ana and Alex decided to get divorced, in a civilized way and remain on good terms, to not hurt Sarah and their families.

At work, Ana did her job like nothing had happened, but the sparkle was gone from her eyes. Most of her coworkers assumed the change had something to do with Ana's daughter, the surgeries, the handicap, the pain.

Nora noticed right away that something wasn't right with her daughter. But she kept it to herself, hoping Ana would open up and tell her what happened—because something had happened, mothers just know. Nora was very sad, but tried to be joyful for Sarah. Poor girl, she didn't need more sadness around her, she had her own.

Ana approached her mom and asked her to have a seat so they could talk. After she finished explaining to her mom what happened between her and Alex, she expected her mom to start talking bad about Alex's behavior. Ana couldn't believe what her mother, her own mother, said.

"Ana, do you remember when I asked you if you make time for your husband, like you make time for your daughter, work, doctors, and physical therapy sessions? And you answered that your mind was only Sarah because of her problems? Well, a mother knows better always. I tried to warn you, but it was useless. Men are different than women; they do need attention from us—doesn't matter what the circumstances are. I know what you are going to answer, so please don't do it. You have to deal with your feelings now. Sarah needs both of you; she needs your love and care. Alex is a good man, and I don't think he's that guilty."

"So, you blame me for what he did? How come I can go to work, take care of everything, take Sarah to her appointments—it is true that he goes with us most of the time—and do my job, plus all the things that come up with Sarah's condition, and I never had a wrong thought in my mind? For me, Alex and Sarah are everything; they are my family. No, I don't want him in my life anymore. I will do it without him. You are right; I have neglected him lately, but it shouldn't make him seek out another woman where he could have 'happy time,' with no problems, no suffering. I thought he was committed to our marriage, but I was wrong. I'm not the first or the last one to have this in her life. Mom, please do not take his side. I'm not totally guilty, and I know it. I need your help, not a lecture. My decision is made."

Nora stopped saying what was in her mind, she took care of her granddaughter, and the day went by like nothing was different from a day before. When she went back to her apartment, she looked a lot older and her body was carrying more pain from her heart. She tried to imagine how Ana's life would be from now on, as a single woman with a handicapped girl that couldn't walk.

"How much can I help? How much can I do, for how long? I'm getting older, my body hurts, my hands hurt, and Ana's divorce will kill me." Nora kept the new situation to herself, the new sad situation.

Sophia loved her mother so much, that she was able to see right away something happened. "Mom, why did you cry? What's happened? Is Sarah ok?"

Of course, her first thought was Sarah. "Sophia, your sister has a problem but she will be ok," Nora explained the situation to her youngest daughter and Sophia's eyes got wider and really sad. She loved her older sister and felt like her problems were her problems, also.

"I think we have to let them solve their problem, and not get involved. We have to wait and see what we can do, but not now."

Nora was very pleased to see Sophia thinking right. It was her thought too. Let them decide their lives; let them have their minds and feelings, and make the decisions they needed for their family, for their daughter, and for themselves.

So, Nora and Sophia would come and play with Sarah, do things around the kitchen to help Ana like nothing happened.

It was one of those days when Sarah and her mom were spending time together, reading and having peace in their minds. Ana was so much into those poems that she didn't pay attention when her husband came home from work. She greeted him politely but cold, with no smile or love. Something caught her eye, something that she didn't want him to know she noticed, but she did. She said, "Are you sick? You scared Sarah and me!"

"I am so sorry; I didn't mean to. I'm ok."

"How can you be ok looking like this? Do you have a fever?" Even though they were separated, they still lived under the same roof. And she did care about him, no matter what.

"Give me a few minutes, and after that, I would like to talk to you, if you want, of course, please."

"Ok," Ana answered. She went back in the kitchen, wondering why her husband, still her husband, looked so bad. She'd never seen him looking like this, a different man, suddenly older! "Why did I accept to talk with him? I'm stupid; I shouldn't talk to him. There's nothing we can talk about. I want to divorce and it is that simple. No, it is not simple at all. We have a child, a handicapped child, and she needs us both." Ana didn't want to talk to Alex, but she was curious to see if he was ready to move out and get the divorce. She didn't really want him to move out because she still loved him, but her pride was making her ask him every day to do so.

Alex came in the kitchen, sat on a chair, and looked at Ana like he was seeing her for the first time. "Is Sarah ok? I promised her we'd watch a movie together today."

"Yes, she's doing ok, but she is struggling with those foot braces. Otherwise, she is doing great."

Alex sat silently for a moment, and then said, "Ana, I love you. I cannot live without you and Sarah. Please take me back and I promise that it will be forever, for the rest of my life."

It was the last thing she expected to hear! She was ready to find out about him moving out and starting a new life with another woman. She wasn't prepared for this, so she didn't answer, just pretended to be busy cooking, like she didn't hear one word. She knew her husband well enough to know that if he would promise something, he would always keep his promises. But she didn't want to share her life with him if he wasn't happy.

Let him be with a woman that will give him happiness, a normal child, a normal life, with no difficult problems like he has with us. He is still with us because he feels obligated, guilted because of Sarah! No, I don't want him back this way. I don't need him. Nothing would ever be the same. No, I do not want him back. Ana still did not answer her husband out loud.

"Ana, please answer! What do you want me to do to prove my intentions, my love? I admit... I tried to have a better life, but nobody, I mean nobody, has your qualities; nobody can be like you. I have always loved you and I always will. I cannot live without you and our daughter. Please forgive me and give me a chance to show you my love? Let me be the man you married. I will never hurt your heart again."

Ana thought about how much her husband was talking. He never talked so much! He must be very hurt. Her mind was so busy thinking of what to say. One thing she knew for sure, she didn't want him back in her life. "Alex, Sarah is waiting for you to watch the movie together."

"Can you answer, please?"

"When Sarah goes to bed, come back here and we can continue our conversation."

"Thank you," he said, grateful he got her talk to him, at least.

Sarah looked so happy to be with her papa. She adored him so much. They had a good time together, and Sarah went to bed with her mom's help.

All that time Alex and Sarah spent together, Ana prayed and talked to God, lifting her heart and tears to him, asking him for advice. She loved her husband, but her feelings were hurt. Yes, she knew she had her part in everything that happened between them. She became calmer with a sense of peace covering her mind.

So, when Alex came back in the kitchen, she said, "Alex, I need time, a lot of time."

"I know it. I love you."

She didn't say one word but 'good night.'

* * * *

Days and nights went by without any change between Ana and Alex. Sarah was all smiles when she wasn't in pain. Her treatments continued, and she did have more surgeries on her tendons and ligaments. Ana was always with her daughter, everywhere she had to go. Alex was taking them for appointments and to the hospitals. The family had dinner together, sharing the events of the day. Looking from the outside, they seemed to be a normal, loving family, but the truth was far different.

Ana dealt with her soul's wounds, trying to forgive. She knew she could forgive, but not forget.

One day, Alex came closer to her, smelling her hair and touching her face, removing a strand of hair that was covering her eyes. The moment she felt his presence close to her body, a warm wave covered her from head to toes. She was melting; her body had been waiting for this for a long time, but she acted like a stone, not letting her feelings show. She distanced herself without saying one word.

Ana tried to fall asleep, but her eyelids couldn't meet. She tossed around and her mind was wondering what the next day would bring. "God, show me the best thing to do for my daughter; she is my love, and she's my life. I love Alex and I'll never love somebody else, but I'm too hurt, too proud to take him back." A dark, heavy cloud, smelling like church incense, covered Ana's mind. She fell asleep thinking that tomorrow would be another day and that God would talk to her, like he always did.

* * * *

Alex had a cousin, a wonderful young lady, married to an amazing man. Together, they had a daughter a few years older than

Sarah. This cousin and her family were close to Alex and his family. They spent many weekends, when they were able to add an extra day to their Sunday, camping together in the mountains. Ana never liked camping, but she loved being with such wonderful people. Sarah was enjoying the fresh mountain air and the company of her cousin. The girls were happy to play and be with each other.

Alex had to carry Sarah everywhere, on the trails, to the river, to the tent. Sarah could say that she saw almost the whole country on her father shoulders!

Ana loved these people very much, feeling like they were a real balm for her soul.

On a recent trip, Ana wanted to get closer to her husband, trying to forgive him. Their love flourished like never before. Alex was patient and waited for his wife to make the first step; he didn't want to hurry things up. Alex knew his wife well. He had to wait for the right time to come. God and only God could show Ana the right decision. Alex said to himself, "I have all the time in the world. I'm not going anywhere. I am here to stay; this is my love, and this is my family."

Not too long after they came back from camping, Alex asked Ana, "Do you know, we're not getting any younger..." Then he stopped saying more. He wanted to continue but he wasn't sure if it was the right moment.

Ana listened to what he said looked confused as to where the conversation was going, what he was trying to say. So he continued speaking, "Ana, did you ever consider having one more child? It would be the best thing we could do for Sarah, to not leave her alone in this world."

Thunder, clouds, lightning, and all kinds of thoughts were storming Ana's head. "Are you insane? How can you even ask such a question? It isn't enough that we have a handicapped child? I am afraid to even think about it. How do you know he or she will be a normal child?"

"Ana, take it easy. Both of us are healthy and still young. You know that what happened to Sarah wasn't our fault. You know it was the doctor's fault. You know all this."

"I know it, but I am scared to death to even think about it."

"Please, let's have some blood tests done, to convince you that I'm right. Hopefully, if you see the results showing what we already know, you will agree."

"I don't know. I don't know," Ana said, crying. She started crying because she had the same thoughts as her husband, but she never said them out loud. She knew this could be her last chance to have another child. Alex hit a very sensitive spot in her heart. "Alex, I've been thinking about this almost every day, but do I have the right to bring an innocent child into this world and put all the responsibilities that come with having a handicapped sister on his or her shoulders? Who gives me this right? Only God has the answer. I am only a granule of sand in this Universe."

Ana and Alex had some complicated blood tests done, and the results came back showing that both of them were perfectly healthy and ready to have another baby. They knew it from the beginning, but Ana needed this for her peace of mind.

But Ana truly knew that God had answered her questions when she became pregnant. Her and Alex had love back in their marriage and it had produced another child. New hopes, new expectations. The whole family celebrated the good news. They all agreed that Sarah needed a brother or a sister, to not be alone later in her life.

* * * *

Sophia married Arthur, her high school sweetheart, and graduated college to become an engineer. Her husband was an architect and, besides his job, he drew cartoons. Sophia's life was a lot better than Ana's. Her father was giving her everything he could, forgetting all the sacrifices Ana made to keep the family above the poverty level. He forgot about the time Ana had to get a full-time job before graduating high school. It seemed like to him, it never happened. Ana never expected something in return for what she did, but she was hurt to see how he continued to make differences between her and his own child. When her stepfather was able to make a good living after he went through hell, he never looked back;

never grateful for Ana's work. Only the love between the sisters kept them together and they never had any arguments, but somewhere inside Ana's heart, it became a wound. Her sister had a much better life, and she did get to go to college. Sophia visited often, though, and enjoyed each moment of her visits. When she heard about her sister being pregnant, she jumped up and down. Sophia hoped one day she would feel the same way as her sister.

Ana was a beautiful pregnant woman. Alex had to do most of the lifting, but still Ana had to care for Sarah, being a woman. The pregnancy was going well, no complications, no problems. When Ana was sitting on a chair, Alex and Sarah would go behind that chair and massage Ana's neck, shoulders, and arms. When the baby inside Ana's stomach would kick, both of them would scream their happiness. They screamed so loud it often scared Ana, but it made her happy to see them touching and talking to the miracle inside her body, her future baby. Just seeing the excitement in their eyes, Ana knew she'd made the right decision to let Alex back in and to have another child.

Sarah kept calling the baby "my little brother" without having any idea if it was a boy or a girl.

When Ana was alone, she talked to her baby. "Son, there is somebody above us, somebody that wants you to take care of your sister, his name is God and he loves you." She realized she said "son" and thought she copied Sarah! It seemed so natural, so normal, to call him 'son,' she thought. Closing her eyes, she prayed and prayed asking God for a normal, healthy baby and a good doctor.

* * * *

"Alex, Alex, wake up, wake up! We have to go to the hospital, hurry up."

It was the third day after the New Year celebration. When they arrived at the hospital, the first thing they heard was the doctor's prediction. "This child will have lots of common sense; he didn't bother anybody on New Year's night. He waited. Nice baby."

Ana smiled and had a good feeling about the place. The doctor was an old university professor, teaching med students. He came closer, looked in Ana's eyes, and said, "I know what you went through with your first child. I am an old-fashioned doctor, and this means that I am going to do a vertical 'C' section, instead of horizontal. This way I will take the baby directly from his cushion with no effort for the baby."

"Doctor, you know better than me. I asked God to bless your hands. I trust you," Ana said, feeling at peace.

"Thank you," the doctor said. "The nurse will be here in a moment."

* * * *

When Ana woke up, the nurse said, "You have the most wonderful, handsome baby I have ever seen!"

"A boy, am I right? Is he ok?"

"Yes, he is doing excellent. What a beautiful baby boy with lots of black hair."

Ana looked up and thanked God for answering her prayers, then fell back to sleep quickly, still feeling the anesthesia's effects.

What a joy! Sarah couldn't wait to hold her brother. "Mom, I want to thank you so much. I will love my brother more than anything in the world, I promise. I will take care of him. I will be like you," she kept saying.

Ana was so happy to see the joy in her daughter's eyes, and she knew Sarah would do everything for her brother, at her level. She would want to play together, but she wouldn't be able to run with him, to do the physical things alongside her brother.

"Ana, I'm the happiest father in the world. I am so glad you decided to have another child. He will make us happier, and he will be a real help for our daughter. Now I know she won't be alone after we are gone. I am so relived. It sounds like we have this child for our own purpose, but it was God's solution for us, and for Sarah."

"I know and I'm happy, too. I cannot believe the joy I saw in Sarah's eyes."

The celebration for the new baby was full of laughter and hope.

All the family members came to celebrate the new addition to the family. Phillip was the name they choose for their son. Ana knew he was healthy and normal, but she couldn't wait to take him for his first check-up, to hear directly from his pediatrician that he was perfect, normal, and healthy.

Ana came home all smiles after the doctor appointment. The results were excellent, and she was dancing with her son in her arms. Sarah was standing in the living room, using a walker, and she joined her mother, moving her body as much as she could.

Anyone could see her joy. Ana's eyes filled with tears seeing the difference, and she knew that from now on, this would be a permanent thing in her mind—the comparison between Sarah and Phillip. But she wouldn't let Sarah see it; not ever. She would teach Phillip to play with his sister the way she could.

Ana was constantly aware of Sarah's reactions to her brother's initiatives, and she was trying to make things easier for Sarah.

"Mom, I would like to run like he does, to play with him," Sarah said. "Not so much for me, but for him, to not slow him down. I see how he always looks behind to see where I am and what I am doing. I keep telling him to go ahead and play, but he always waits for me. I'm so sorry for him. I feel like sometimes I am an obstacle for him."

"How can you talk like this? He loves you more than he loves me! Can't you see it? He wants to wait for you; he wants to be with you."

"I know, but I see how he plays with the kids his age. It is such a difference."

"Don't compare how he plays with you and how he plays with the other children. You're his sister, and he adores you. He knows already that you are special, and you are my sunshine—you're my life, my love…you are my reason for existing."

"Mom, how can you say these kinds of things? What about Phillip? H's your son, my brother; you should love him the same way, if not more."

"Sarah, I know this and you're perfectly right. I love your brother with all my heart, but there is something special, different in my love for you."

"Because of my handicap, because I cannot walk?"

"I don't know. I have no answer. All I know is that my love for you has no words to be explained and only the facts can reflect what I am trying to say. I would give my life for the both of you, but when I look at you, I feel like I need one more life to do everything I would like to do for you."

Phillip was growing fast, and he became an amazing, good-looking boy. Black eyes, black hair, and white beautiful skin were Phillip's best features. He was tall for his age, smart and curious. He wanted to know everything. When his time came to crawl, he was the funniest thing anyone could see. He was crawling backwards! Phillip enjoyed crawling backwards and he loved "parking" between the legs of any chair that was closest to him. He was "parking" perfectly. Actually, he loved playing with cars, trucks, and anything else that had wheels. If somebody would give him a car, he was the happiest child in the world, for a few hours, of course.

Sarah loved listening to music, so the music was on every single moment in their apartment, and this made Phillip very happy. He would hold on to everything he could to keep himself up, and he would dance all day long. What an exercise! Sarah noticed how much her brother loved the music, so she already knew what songs he liked. They had fun together, and their parents were so grateful to see their kids' love for each other.

Sophia and her husband came to visit and spend time with their nephew and niece.

Sarah was fourteen years old already, not a kid anymore, but she liked to be called a kid, because she felt closer to her brother.

"Ana, soon, we are going to leave Romania, as you know, but I'm devastated thinking of what I leave behind," Sophia said.

Ana knew the things her sister and her brother-in-law were going through. They applied to leave the country and live in the USA, and this was considered a crime! Arthur had published some political cartoons mocking the Communist Party. Ana had no idea how he was able to publish these cartoons, but he did. They were so young, had no children, but they had dreams. Both of them wanted to live in America; they were dreaming of all the things they could accomplish living in a free country. They loved that country and were thinking of it every single second. Arthur knew there would be consequences and he would be in trouble if he published those cartoons, but he wanted to be in trouble. He wanted to be free and his wife had the same feelings. His actions brought him the trouble he was looking for, but at the same time, brought the blessings he dreamed of—he got a call from the USA embassy to come for an interview!

The gift of his life, his dreams were getting closer. Sophia and Arthur received the approval of the USA to live there. Both of them had college educations and they were so young, so full of hopes and dreams.

The family was sad, but everybody understood and approved their actions. It was like they were thinking: if I could, I would leave this country, too. But it wasn't the country, it was the regime—the Communists, the economy, the situation they were living in. People were free without the freedom. They couldn't travel to see other countries, to see their friends! For most of them, it was like living in a free prison, a beautiful, magnificent prison with mountains, the Black Sea, monasteries, castles, the Danube, and amazing old cities full of history. Everywhere you went, you could see the history of the country marking every place. You could see all the stamps of history, triggering a feeling of pride for being part of so much culture and tradition.

Sophia's heart was broken; she knew it would be hard to say goodbye, but she never believed it would be this hard. All day long, she had tears in her eyes, but it was something she dreamed of and she was so young. It was almost like she had to try to have a better life, to not live under the Communist regime. Her husband learned English in school, and Sophia was practicing the language every day, knowing she would get a job in America, and she wanted to do well from the beginning. Sophia tried to convince Ana that she had to apply to leave the country for medical reasons, so Sarah could have a better life.

Ana knew very well how much care the handicapped people had in America. She'd read so much about it in foreign magazines, which were prohibited in Romania. Ana had a friend that worked at a duty-free shop at the airport, so she had access to French and American newspapers and magazines. It was common sense and pretty easy to understand why the government didn't let people travel as they could see how other people lived, really being free! Ana promised her sister she would look into it, and that she would start applying for the American visa for her whole family.

When Sophia left the country, it was a devastating day for Nora and Ana, but they both had hope that the young couple would be much better off living in America. Things were getting harder and harder for Sarah to cooperate due to her physical handicap, because the regime wasn't interested in doing anything for these people, considering them to be a shame for the government and for the country. What a mentality! It was because of the money the regime would have to spend to improve those people's lives. It was the only reason. Their money had to go into grandiose palaces and huge buildings to fit their taste of opulence and ugliness.

Ana remembered when her parents' homes were leveled by bulldozers and how the Communists built villas and different types of huge mansions for the members of the Communist Party, to be closer to downtown, to live centrally. Too many painful memories; too many things dear to her heart had been leveled, too. Ana shook her head and tried to forget about all these things; they were too painful and she'd had enough pain in her heart for two lifetimes!

* * * *

Sophia and Arthur arrived in America as political refugees and they were taken care of. Being highly educated and speaking the language, it was relatively easy to get situated. They both got good jobs and started living a real, good life. Sophia was missing her family so much that she called once a week. She was able to convince her sister to start the papers for immigration.

Sophia and her husband never found out what happened before they left the country and what Alex had been told to do, which he refused, and how proud Ana was of her husband for refusing to be an obstacle for Sophia's new life.

Alex's position at work was a very good one; he was very appreciated. But once his sister-in-law left the country, his position became "unhealthy!"

It was unacceptable to be in such a good position and have relatives who left the country to live in a capitalist country. Alex had been advised by one of his superiors to go to the department that issued passports and fill out a special form showing his opposition for his sister-in-law's departure. By filling out such a document, he could be "covered" and his job would be stable.

Alex came home and explained to his wife what his boss had told him to do in order to keep his job. They couldn't believe how mean those people were and how low they were willing to play to keep their protection from the Communist Party.

"Ana, if I had signed that document, and I am sure they asked your cousins to do the same thing, but they were afraid to talk, your sister would have never left the country. You know my answer. I never agreed to sign such an atrocity, such a horrible condemnation. I refused to say yes; I refused to go and sign the paper. Who am I to kill their dreams? I have no right to do it. I know I'm responsible for my family and for my two children, but I couldn't do it. Ana, God will take care of us. I know it."

Ana agreed with her husband's decision and both knew from that moment on, his job would be in jeopardy, that he could be jobless soon. They knew it.

Alex knew that he would be treated differently and his action would have severe consequences. One, and the most important, was losing his job. He worked so hard to bring honor to his country by training Olympic champions and creating a solid sport department at the college where he worked, with promising results. Ana's sister never found out what her brother-in-law did for her—she was always the lucky one.

Alex waited for the children to go to bed and asked Ana to come closer so they could listen to the "forbidden" Voice of America! It was the highlight of their days, besides the fun they had with Phillip. It was the only radio broadcast to tell them what was going on in the world. Hiding behind closed doors, afraid to be heard by the neighbors, almost everybody had the same routine. It was their refuge, to listen to the Western world, and it was really dangerous to do it. Alex and Ana were so tired of their national newspapers and radio stations that were dedicated to the Communist Party and all the "wonderful" things done for the benefit of the people. What a joke! Twenty-four hours the only thing you could hear about was about the leader of the Party. People hated him. He was a dictator that had ruined so many lives, keeping the country in poverty. The only good thing that party ever achieved was the education. It was true that students had to go six days every week to school, but the results were amazing. Romanian students were leading European school contests, winning gold medals, daily.

* * * *

Over the course of a year, Sophia was calling her sister once a week, insisting she should convince the family to leave Romania and come live in America.

Alex realized how much better it would be to live in a country where handicapped people were treated with respect and care, where being disabled wasn't a shame!

Ana was already convinced that they would have to make the move, to help her daughter to become independent, to live a normal life. She knew Sarah would have a much better future. She started dreaming, seeing her daughter going to college and meeting people who shared common interests. This was a huge decision to make— they were deciding their children's future! They were concerned about their family, though, knowing that their decision would put a bad mark on their jobs—the same thing that happened when Sophia left the country.

So, one day, husband and wife grabbed the bull by the horns and entered the USA embassy, located in the middle of the city. They knew that the moment they made the first step behind the building fence, their jobs would be lost. They knew that everybody would find out in minutes, not hours. They were aware of the consequences, the "punishments" that were coming their way.

Ana's work place was an institute for the chemical industry, a headquarters. The leader of the institute was the dictator's wife! Ana knew, the next day, her job would be gone. If she worked in a modest place, maybe it would take a little bit longer to be fired, but working in such a "prestigious" place, they wouldn't tolerate a bad example for all the employees. She would be considered a traitor and unacceptable to work there.

Ana was right...they had good spies. And they found out fast about Ana's request to leave the country.

"Ana, the boss wants to see you in his office, now."

"Ok, I will be there in a moment." She opened the door and her boss started talking, without greeting her or inviting her to sit down. Ana knew her boss was a good, Christian man, because they shared some thoughts together when nobody could hear their conversation, but he had to protect his position. He was a solid member of the Communist Party. Ana was prepared to hear the sentence; she knew almost word by word what was next. She understood her boss' situation...he had to do his job, he had to keep his job. So she listened to everything he had to say, being polite and calm.

"Ana, we consider you a traitor. Your actions made us decide to let you go, now in this moment. You are not allowed to go back to your office. Somebody will bring your belongings, and you are asked to leave the institute's property right away. You're going to receive the money we owe you for the time you have worked. One of my assistants will escort you outside the institute."

Ana tried to justify her boss's behavior. *Not even a goodbye, maybe he was afraid of microphones in his office?* She waited a few minutes outside the office and soon after that, was escorted to the gate. Somebody she didn't know brought her purse and the few things she had in her drawers. She wasn't even allowed to say goodbye to the coworkers she'd worked with for so many years. Twenty-seven years! Those people were her work family; she had been so appreciated as a human being and for her professional skills. Ana was one of the best employees, even though she never enrolled in the Communist Party. She'd always found an excuse to not become a member. She had no chance to tell him that she applied to leave the country for medical reasons, for her daughter's sake. All the way home, Ana was shaking and crying.

"Mom, I am so glad you came home!" Sarah said.

Seeing Sarah without Phillip was unusual for Ana; typically, by the time she was getting home from work, both children were home, waiting for Alex and her. So, for a few moments she forgot about her problem and Phillip came to her mind. She adored her son; she would give her life for him. Phillip had started at the elementary school, and he was doing much better than in the kindergarten. Ana didn't know why she suddenly remembered Phillip's reactions to the place she took him, every morning. Phillip hadn't liked going to the kindergarten. In fact, he'd hated it. Every time he would write with his left hand, the teacher would hit him with a wooden ruler, saying he had to write with his right hand. Poor child! He couldn't hold the pen in his right hand; he was a lefty, but the government said that everybody had to write with the right hand...never use the left hand.

Ana remembered how many times she had to go to the kindergarten to pick her son up and bring him home. Phillip hated going to his kindergarten so much that he was getting a fever when Ana dropped him there. The doctor explained to her that it was a 'mechanical fever' caused by stress. She'd never heard about it before, but the facts proved the doctor's diagnosis. Phillip was doing better in school because the teacher didn't hit him, letting him write with his left hand even as she insisted he use the right one.

"Hi, my dear, let me hug you."

"What's happened. Why did you come home so early?" Nora asked her daughter. "Are you ok? Are you sick?"

"No, Mom, I am ok. I got fired because of the application we made at the USA embassy."

"What? You just did it! How is this possible?"

"I know it, but the government is a lot faster than we think they are. I wonder how long it will take for Alex to be fired. I have to start asking all our friends to help us to find jobs, anywhere, anything, only to bring money home. But everybody will be scared to help us, to avoid being punished for helping traitors. I expected this to happen but not so soon; it happened way too soon."

"Let me call Peter. He has always helped us. He is the one to call. Do you remember how he helped us when we had to have you working?"

"Yes, unfortunately, I do remember that. I will never forget I couldn't go to college. You shouldn't remind me about that horrible time in my life, at least not now— but it is ok, I love you, Mom. I will always love you."

They hugged each other with tears in their eyes. The past hurt so much and it seemed the present wasn't too far from hurting them again.

"Mom, please, let's wait for Alex to come home. I want to be sure we don't have to ask for two jobs. At the same time, I don't want Peter to have problems helping us. He has a high position now; he is the director of a big manufacturer and he is also a member of the Communist Party. I'm afraid he cannot help us. You noticed I didn't say he doesn't want to help. I know him so well, but he can't put his job in danger for helping us. I don't want something to happen to him because of us."

"You're right. Let's wait and see how things go."

"I think we should ask friends first, the ones that don't have anything to do with the Communist Party."

Nora knew what her job was—Ana and Alex had to find work, to take care of their children, to put food on the table. Who knows how long it would take to receive the American visa? Even then, they didn't know exactly what their future will be.

Alex came home from work, and when he heard about Ana's job, he asked the same question as his mother-in-law. "How could that be possible, so fast? How did they find out that quickly? They have their own people working there and they spy for them, for sure. Ana, don't worry. We'll find something to make money. I still have my job."

Nora called her nephew as soon as she got home. "Peter, can you come and have lunch with me? I have something very important to talk to you about and I cannot talk on the phone. You know why." She knew how dangerous it would be for Peter to help his cousin, but at the same time, she knew how much love there was between Ana and her cousins. They grew up like siblings in the same home, same place, until their homes were leveled by the Communists.

Peter came to Nora's apartment and they shared memories and had a good time together. He made time to be with his favorite aunt. Peter wasn't surprised to hear about Ana's job. Everybody expected this to happen, but not so fast. He knew how hard it would be for his cousin to be accepted for work anywhere because of her new status…a traitor that asked to leave the country! Nobody would even listen to him, but he always helped her. He would never forget the promise he made when Ana's father committed suicide. Being the older cousin, he promised to always take care of Ana and he'd kept his promise so far. He knew Ana would do the same thing for him and his children, no matter what the circumstances were. The love for his family was bigger and more important than his job.

Nora was almost shocked when her nephew said, "Aunt Nora, tomorrow morning, I will talk to some of my friends, especially one of my coworkers that thinks like I do. I have no other choice."

"Yes, you can say no," Nora said.

"Aunt Nora, you know better than me that I will never say no when it is about my family. I will find something for Ana and keep your fingers crossed that nobody will find out that I helped her. I can lose my job and you know it."

"Thank you from the bottom of my heart for helping Ana to find a job. Thank you and God bless you and your family."

* * * *

Alex still had no problems at his work place, and they couldn't be more thankful for this. He didn't hear anybody talking about his application to leave the country and everything seemed to be like usual.

Peter talked to his friends that worked in different places and asked them to help him to find a job, any kind of job, for his cousin who had two children. He knew who he could talk to. There were people like him, working hard but hating the regime. These people understood each other without saying much. Ana was lucky. Peter was able to locate a factory that needed workers. One of Peter's friends was the director of that factory and he wanted to help his friend. Peter couldn't wait to bring the good news to his cousin. "Ana, I got you a job! But the job is in a factory."

"Oh my God, thank you, thank you so much. How did you know I needed a job? My mother talked to you? Am I right?"

"Don't be silly; who cares? You have a job; that's all that counts."

"I have a job. I have a job! Peter, I will be so grateful for the rest of my life. You could lose your job for what you did for me."

"I will do anything for you and your family. We are like brother and sister. You did the right thing by applying to leave the country. You did it for your daughter. You have all the reasons in the world to want to help her to have a better life. I would do the same thing for my children if I had a situation like yours. Ok, now I have to work and I'll see you soon. I love you, Ana."

"I love you forever and I will call my mom to let her know."

Nora already knew about the job. She was so proud of herself that she asked her nephew right away and didn't wait for things to become facts.

Ana was screaming when her husband came home. "Alex, I got a job!"

"What? How? Who helped you to find a job?"

"Guess. Who do you think could do this for us?"

"Peter."

"You see, you are right. He put his job in danger to help us." Ana was ready to start working at her new work place. She never worked in a factory, but she knew she would do her best and the coworkers would love her like all others she had. She started working there and she was so right. It was a different environment but the people were the same; they were the ones creating the atmosphere. She was surrounded by good people, helping her to get adjusted with her new position. Ana was a quick learner and soon ,she became a reliable worker.

Alex was participating at one of the Communist Party meetings.

A long time ago, he had to become a member in order to obtain his job. His position couldn't be covered by somebody that did not belong to the Communist Party. It was considered unsafe to teach students or to coach sports men if you were not indoctrinated with the Communist ideology. He had to accept it, to get and to keep his job.

"Alex, you have to be in the boss's office at 11:00 a.m.," a coworker said.

"What's wrong?" he asked. The coworker had no idea about Alex's application. Nobody knew, because Alex didn't want his friends to suffer from knowing the truth. "Ok, thank you. I will go."

Alex opened the door and his boss was looking at him like was seeing him for the first time.

"Alex, starting tomorrow you won't be working here anymore. What in the world did you do? I received instructions to let you go and I couldn't ask why. An order is an order and as you know, we don't ask; we execute it."

"Sir, I requested to leave the country and I filled out an application for the USA visa."

"What did you just say? Do you want to leave the country? Are you insane? When did you do this?"

"Last month, sir," Alex answered.

"And they let you work here for the whole month? Something must be wrong, because, normally, you apply today and they fire you yesterday."

"Sir, I have a handicapped child in a wheelchair, and I have to think of her future, to see her living independently."

"I understand, and I am so sorry to hear about this. I wish you the best in your new adventure. Please, listen to what I was told to tell you: You are not allowed to be in contact with any of our students or the staff of the university. Go get your things and your payment will be sent to your home, or you can come to the financial office and get it, but without communicating with any of the members. I cannot say much, but I wish you good luck."

"Thank you, sir, I was happy working here." Alex gathered his things, said goodbye to a few people that were around him, and went home. His heart was as heavy as a stone. So many memories, so many achievements, so much hard work. All those students he trained, some became champions, and some became teachers or coaches. He tried to eliminate those thoughts from his mind, but it was hard.

"Hi, Alex," Nora said. "Coming home earlier means you got fired, am I right?"

"Yes, my turn came; you learn your lesson."

"I cannot wait to see Ana's face when she finds out you lost your job, even if she expected this to come. But, do you know something? Everything will be just fine. Look at Ana, she has a job now; and you will find one, for sure."

Ana came home and as soon as she saw her husband home, earlier than normal, she knew what had happened. She was calm, and without letting him say anything, she said, "Alex, I work with a young woman whose father is the director of the transportation department for the Jewish Federation."

"What does this have to do with our situation?" Alex asked, having no clue.

"It does. Tomorrow, I will talk to her and she will talk to her father to help us, to find you a job."

"Why do think she will want to help us?"

"She's a woman with a big heart and she likes me very much."

"Oh, let's hope and pray she will get something for me, anything. I will do anything."

The next morning, Ana talked to her young coworker and asked if she could do something to help them. The coworker was so excited to be able to do something for Ana. She had so much respect for Ana that she considered her a mentor, learning a lot from Ana's experience.

The money Ana was paid for her job was a lot less than she had before, but Ana felt so grateful to have it. All the food was rationed; they had coupons for so much butter, meat, flour, sugar, oil. Everything was portioned and you couldn't find food on the shelves. The electricity, the gas, the food, everything was rationed. Phillip had to watch outside and let his family know when the "food truck" came, so they could run and stand in line to get their food. The apartment building was right behind the shopping center where the grocery store was located. Phillip learned how to play "waiting for the food truck," and all his friends were doing the same thing. Those kids were way too young to realize how sad their games were, but at the same time, they were helping their families to get food. The lines were long and people were stepping on each other to get to the counter, to be sure they got their "portions." The family had a tough time, but no worse than anybody around them.

People belonging to the Communist Party, among the higher ranks, were doing really well. They had all the necessary things and a lot more. They had huge mansions, unbelievable vacations, nice clothes, good food, everything.

Ana had decided long ago to never envy those people, as she would never do what they were doing, to pretend you love what you hate the most!

Ana's friend and coworker asked her father to help Ana's husband and to try to find him something for work. After a few days, Alex had a job interview at the Jewish Federation. The interview went really well and he was offered a driver position. He accepted right away, happy to have a job.

"Ana, we are going to celebrate. I got a job. I'm so happy."

Nobody asked what kind of job it was. They were just grateful he would be bringing money home. He started driving a van that had meals inside for the older Jewish people. He didn't handle the food—he wasn't Jewish—but he drove the people in charge to the homes of the people receiving the meals.

Things were getting settled, job-wise. Every day was filled with school, work, and family time, but Ana realized how long it was taking to receive the approval for the green card from the American embassy. She wrote a letter explaining the family's situation, Sarah's condition, and all the details she considered the consul would need to evaluate their case.

When Phillip got home from school, she took him with her and walked together around the embassy for hours.

Poor guy, he couldn't understand why they had to walk in cold, snow, rain, or heat, but he was happy to join his mother. Ana was walking up and down, restless, knowing and hoping somebody would call her inside, one day.

After a week passed, she made an appointment to see a representative of the American embassy and to give them one more letter.

CHAPTER THIRTEEN

Five years, for five full years, it went on like that. Alex and Ana took turns going to the embassy, and they never gave up hope. They knew that one day they would live in America.

One day, during Ana's walks at the embassy, somebody approached her and invited her inside. It was an icy, cold day but Ana's heart was hot and beating fast. She was introduced to a nice, tall gentleman that invited her to sit down.

He started talking about her case, calmly and softly, he said, "Ana, imagine your home is America and you would like to invite people to your home for dinner. How many people can you invite? The answer is: You can invite as many people you have room and food for, so those people will be taken care of and they will have what they need to feel comfortable and safe. So, you have to wait for your turn to come, your invitation to dinner. I hope you understand, and I want you to know how impressed I am by your persistence, your desire to live in my country. You're going to be a very good citizen; I know it. It was nice seeing you again, because I see you all the time through the window."

Ana thanked the gentleman and left, feeling sure they would never be "invited to dinner" because of Sarah's condition. There were so many other people that applied a long time after they did and they had already left and were living in America.

Five years of hopes, five years of punishments, five years of marching quiet and peacefully holding her son's hands and hiding all the papers in her bra. She knew she could be arrested if somebody would read what she wrote to the consul. She was disappointed, but she didn't give up.

"Did you go again? You will never give up, am I right?" Alex asked his wife.

"Yes, and you should know better by now what kind of wife you chose. We are good people, we can become successful and you know what? We will. Tomorrow, you know where to find me and your son. I feel so sorry for him to learn each stone of that street, but I'm inventing games so he is learning something new every time we go there."

Thinking about not giving up, Ana remembered a conversation she typically had with her husband when he was still coaching and traveling with his team for European competitions.

"Ana, soon I will go to Austria for an important competition. Every time I go to a Western country, I ask you if you want me to ask for political asylum and stay there till we can be reunited. So, what do you think?"

"Alex, you know my answer. You do what you want to do, but I believe in leaving the country all or none. Who knows how long it would take to be reunited? Maybe you are right, maybe it would be a lot faster that way, but I prefer to leave our country legally and together as a family."

"Ok. Don't say that I didn't ask you, just as I do every time I go somewhere where I could obtain political asylum. If you change your mind, let me know; we still have a few more days till my departure. The most important thing is that I live for you and for our children and I love you so much."

"I know it and I promise I will think about it and let you know."

Those conversations were one of the first things Alex mentioned to his wife when he'd found out he was fired. "Ana, do you remember when I would ask you about political asylum and how you answered? It is ok. You're right. We're together, and I really feel better this way."

Ana remembered all those conversations regarding leaving the country.

Sometimes she felt guilty that she didn't say yes! You can ask for political asylum after you arrive, and then already be in the country when the approval goes through.

Sometimes she felt sorry that she hadn't let him decide by himself about leaving the country, but she always considered it wiser to be together. Her husband kept proving her right.

"Look what I brought home," Alex said, smiling.

"Oh, where did you get all these? Our neighbors will think we are rich!" Ana exclaimed. "Are you crazy? This is really good, quality food. I am so happy. Now we can save our coupons for another time. Phillip, you don't have to watch for the food truck for a week! Alex, tell me, please, how in the world were you able to get all these?"

Phillip thought his mom was crazy and he couldn't understand how somebody could be so happy to see food! It was only food.

"Well, I was put on the list by the Jewish Federation and from now on, we're going to have food, good food. We can even help our families. What a blessing!"

* * * *

The next day, when Nora came to take care of Sarah, Ana opened the door smiling and happy. She couldn't stop thinking how beautiful her daughter looked. She was convinced they received the green card.

"Mom, look what Alex brought home from work! I am so happy."

"Who gave him all these? Why?"

"The Jewish Federation, where he works and we are going to get it on a regular basis from now on. They put him on their list."

Suddenly, Nora's face lit up with a big smile. Nora remembered when Maria, her older sister, helped their Jewish neighbors by hiding them in the basement of their home during the Nazi raids. She remembered how brave she'd been when she went outside and confronted the Nazi soldiers looking for Jewish people, to take them to special death camps. The soldiers had a warrant to check the house. Among the Nazi soldiers, there were some of their own neighbors that adhered to the Nazi army, to protect their families and to survive. Maria had helped most of their wives deliver their babies. Maria did an unforgettable thing; she was so brave and fearless. She could have been killed or arrested right there in front of her house. The Nazis had no mercy, but the soldiers, those knowing what she did for their families, left and they never came back to check Maria's house.

They knew there were Jewish people there! Maria saved so many lives, and Nora realized that what happened to her daughter had a connection with the past. "Ana, I want you to know this. I never put these things together, but today, something struck me like lightning! Years ago, before you were born, we went through a war and the Nazi army were arresting Jewish people." She told Ana the entire story, then ended it with the connection she just made. "What happened to you and your family, the fact that you found help, jobs, and food from the Jewish Federation, when the whole country lives in misery, is a return of blessings for what your aunt did! I strongly believe this."

"Thank you, Mom, for sharing your memories with me. I wish I knew more. Maybe, sometime, we'll sit down and you can tell me more. It is fascinating to find out what happened many years ago. I wish I knew more about my grandparents, about my own father. I was only seven years old when he left from this planet. Mom, I cannot even say that I miss him because I didn't get to know him as a human being, but I do miss him as my father. I feel like I never had a father. It is so sad. Sometimes, when I look back at my married life, I realize how much I wanted my kids to have their own father, not a stepfather, and how that could happen in a heartbeat."

"I know, Ana. You did the right thing. Alex is an amazing father, and he adores you. Your decision was the right one. I wasn't as wise as you."

"Mom, I know what you mean. Do not blame yourself that you married Nick, my stepfather. You were so scared of the future; you were so afraid you couldn't make it. It is ok with me now. Look what a beautiful and smart daughter you have, and I am not talking about me." Ana laughed. "Sophia turned out to be on our side. She doesn't look at all like her father and this makes me happy. I better stop talking because I am mean!"

Mother and daughter hugged each other with tears in their eyes. Ana had so much love and respect for her mother, and these feelings would follow her all her life.

* * * *

People started giving Ana so many compliments for the way she dressed herself, thinking she had a high salary or a husband working for the government. They had no idea that all the clothes and other good things were coming from the Jewish Federation!

One day, Ana came home from work and told Alex, joking, "We are doing so well now that we should stay here and forget about America!"

Alex couldn't believe what he heard. He thought she was serious, but then he looked at her and realized she was laughing.

"Oh Alex, I cannot wait to be approved, to get the green card, and to start a new life. To see Sarah independent and doing things that are impossible here. Nobody wants to leave their country and live in a foreign country with different language, different culture, nobody—but we have to. Our daughter will thank us later for our sacrifice. I'm not so sure about Phillip. He is strong, healthy and he could do well here like all our family did, but it seems like he was born with a mission. Sometimes, I feel sorry for him having such a load on his shoulders, from his birth. But they are siblings, and they love each other a lot. This makes my heart happy. Looking back, I know we made the right decision, and it is not only about our son, you know what I am trying to say."

"Ana, I do know. I love you. Nothing in this world can stop us from getting the best for Sarah and for our handsome son. When I take him for a walk, people stop to touch him and say how beautiful he is. I always answer that he looks like his mama! They smile, and I smile too, because I know I'm a good-looking guy, but seriously, he does look like you."

"I agree," Ana said, very satisfied with her husband's answer as she laughed teasing him. "Speaking of our green card, I do believe somebody will pay attention to our case and I truly believe that we will get it. We'll go to America; you will see."

Going to the American embassy became like a part-time job for Ana. Security officers, clerks, cleaning personnel, consuls, all knew her and her son. Not even bad weather could stop her from going there each week.

One day, while she was "marching" quietly up and down the embassy floors, she remembered another incident in their life that could have cost Alex his life or his freedom. Suddenly, she felt guilty that she hadn't mentioned it on the letter she wrote to the American consul. "How could I be that stupid? How did I miss the most important event that could bring us the approval, the green card?"

Just before Alex was fired for political reasons, he came home and told Ana, "I resigned from the Communist Party. I am not a member anymore."

"No, this is impossible. Nobody ever heard of such a thing. This is a bad joke, Alex; don't do this to me, please?"

"Ana, I did it. This isn't a joke. I couldn't take it anymore."

"Why did you do this? Now they are going to find a way to kill you—a car could hit you when you cross the street! Who knows what they are capable of doing? You should know a lot better than me. I was never a member of that party."

"What will be, will be," Alex had said and started playing with Phillip.

Ana remembered that Alex's resignation made headlines! The very next day, the newspapers talked about Alex, denigrating him, using ugly words, saying that he wasn't worthy to be part of the Communist Party. She came home from the embassy and started doing things around the house. At the time, she had no idea what her husband had done. His resignation from the Communist Party could open the doors of the American embassy!

She checked the mailbox religiously, hoping for a response. It didn't take long.

The mailboxes were in the lobby of the apartment building. She went to pick up the day's mail and noticed the American embassy address. Her hands shook and all the other envelopes between her hands fell on the floor.

"Oh, thank you, God! Thank you, God," she said over and over, all the way to the first floor, where they lived.

Her mom was there, helping with the kids. When she saw her daughter's face full of happiness, she realized something major must have happened.

"Mom, we got the visa! They approved us to live there! This is the visa; this is the visa. And this is the green card. Six years—six years and now finally, we got it. I couldn't be happier than this." Ana started crying.

Her mom came over to her, crying for her daughter, crying tears of happiness. "Ana, this is one of the happiest days of my life—to see you happy and to see how close you are to seeing your own daughter achieve an independent status. Now, I am going to have two daughters in the USA! I am going to pack my luggage," she joked.

Sarah was reading a book when her mom entered the room. "Close your eyes. I have something for you," Ana said to her.

Sarah was afraid that something bad had happened, but looking at her mom's face, she saw the happy smile so she was happy, too. "Mom, please, tell me what happened."

"Sarah, my love, we will go to America! There are so many things to talk about. You will be so much better living there. America cares about people that cannot walk or see, or that have any other handicap; they do a lot for those people. There are sidewalks, ramps for wheelchairs, buses, and so much more that we don't even know about. One thing I know for sure. We are going to start a new, better life, soon. It took us six years, but we got it. Your father doesn't know yet; he is at work. I cannot wait to tell him."

"I cannot wait to see Papa's face when you tell him about the letter."

Always her papa. Ana knew that her children, both of them, loved their father more than they loved her. She remembered one day, Alex was holding his son in his arms and Ana asked Phillip for something, she didn't remember what it was, and her son refused to give it to her. So, Ana said, "Phillip, I am your mother, please, give it to me."

"No, my father is my mother."

Ana had been speechless, but extremely happy to see her kids loving their father so much.

Ana was waiting for Alex to get home. She knew he was picking up Phillip from school. When he finally got home, the first thing he said was, "We are home; we are hungry!"

Ana jumped up and hugged both of them at the same time, so hard that it almost hurt Phillip.

"Mom, what's happened?"

"Son, we are going to America! America! I am so happy."

Alex had tears in his eyes as he looked up and made the cross sign, thanking God. "What a relief! So much joy, so much happiness. What did Sarah say?"

"She's thinking of all our relatives more than thinking of herself. This is going to be the toughest thing to do, to say goodbye. I will be really busy from now on. There will be so many things to take care of, getting organized, paperwork. And I have no idea where to start from."

"What about dinner?" Alex tried to calm her down.

"Who can eat now?"

"Me and the kids. Ana, we will have plenty time to do everything. Nobody will take our visa back. Let's eat first."

Ana realized he was right and tried to serve dinner, but her mind was already planning, organizing, packing. They had one of the happiest dinners they ever had! And not because of the food, but because of the hope.

"Ana, get ready to cry a lot. We have to say goodbye to so many relatives, friends, coworkers, and neighbors."

"I know it, but I cannot let the tears slow me down. I have to be strong. Our life is just beginning. I know we're going to leave a huge part of our hearts here—where we were born—and we have an earthly connection that is undeniable. Thank God, I have my kids to keep me busy, so it will be a little bit easier. At least, I hope so."

"They're my kids, too," Alex joked.

"I know, but I am the mother!"

"Not true! Do you remember when you tried to convince Phillip that he has to love you more because you are his mother? Do you remember his answer?"

"Unfortunately, I do. He answered, 'No, my father is my mother!' How could I ever forget this answer? He was so young and it hurt me a lot, but I am so happy seeing how much both of them love you."

"Ok. Now that we laughed a little, let's get to work. Grab a notebook and write down what we have to do every day."

"I'm determined to do the best for our new life. I pray for God to give us strength to do his work, because this is only his work. Oh, and one more thing Alex. Do you remember that day when those two women from the government asked me to give up our daughter, saying that it was a shame to have a handicapped child? Saying that her problems would keep me away from being professional, productive, that I would need too many medical, sick days, and have too many expenses. Do you remember that day? Well, every time I miss my country, that will be my medication to feel better…remembering that day."

"Of course, I remember, Ana. How can ever I forget it? Let me hug you, please, stop crying. We're going to be ok. It will be hard, new beginning, but full of freedom and hopes. Let's start thinking and write down a plan."

* * * *

The big day came. The large group formed by their relatives and friends was taking up a big space of the waiting area in the airport. Hugs, tears, lots of tears, well wishes, kisses, and so much emotion. Chris was celebrating his birthday that day and the coincidence was too much for both of them. It was a celebration with tears and hopes. He knew how much moving to America meant for Sarah, and he knew how much better she would be living there, but his love for Ana was so deep.

All the family and friends who came to say goodbye had to give them the final goodbye kiss.

The journey was finally beginning. Tears ran down everybody's cheeks, waving their hands in the air, following them with their eyes.

A huge plane took the happy family to their new destination, a place where God sent them to live.

* * * *

"Where in the world have sixteen hours gone? It seemed like only a second.

Sixteen hours of flying, with a short break in Munich, Germany." Ana looked through the windows of the airplane, thinking that the only part missing from their new "puzzle" was their family. It would be really hard to live without them after spending all their lives together, but Ana tried to encourage herself, visualizing the new life. But thousands of doubts started circulating in her mind.

Am I insane to go to America with two children, one in a wheelchair, and I'm the only one who speaks English? And you had six years to think about this, why now? Because I am scared. It is such a huge change; it is the unknown. Sighing at her fears and doubts, she covered her daughter and looked at her son. They slept peacefully, but Alex was watching her.

Yes, he knew exactly what was going on in his wife's mind. They smiled and were encouraging each other by just looking into each other's eyes. He had the same fears, the same thoughts.

The plane could have flown on their energy, on their desires to start a new life. The plane landed at JFK Airport, and in that moment, it felt like blessings were pouring from the sky. Their sponsor was a famous international organization responsible for helping political refugees, to get them settled in. They went through customs and had their documents stamped. Somebody was waiting for them and some other families that arrived on the same flight. A long van was waiting to take all the families and drop them at their designated addresses. Ana and her family were dropped in front of an apartment building located in Brooklyn, New York. It was around 10:00 p.m. It was late, and they were exhausted but happy.

The driver of the van helped them get their stuff from the van and handed Alex a map and a ten-dollar bill. "Tomorrow, twelve o'clock sharp, you have to be at this address. Do not be late. Good luck to all of you." He left without another word.

They started to get closer to the building. Alex pushed the button, and shortly after, a young man came and opened the door to let them in. He introduced himself as the superintendent of the building, let them inside, and took them to their apartment. It was located on the first floor and was a lot more spacious than what they had back home.

Three mattresses were on the floor alongside a TV.

The superintendent said, "I am glad you are here. I live next door to you. If you need something, just ring the bell and I will be more than happy to help you. Good night."

"What a nice man," Ana said after the superintendent left the apartment.

They started unpacking, looking for clothes to wear for the meeting. The family hugged and kissed each other, and soon the children were asleep. Ana and Alex opened the subway map they got from the driver.

Ana said, "I know I'm a city girl, but not this kind of city! This one is huge and a lot bigger than I thought, so how are we going to find the address? How are we going to get there? Alex, you're the expert; check the map and I know you will figure it out."

"Ok, let me see it." What a feeling! He felt tired, very tired, but full of hope and dreams. He spread the map on the floor, looked at it for few minutes, and then told Ana, "Tomorrow morning, we have to go to the subway station; actually, we are right here, the end of the line. Take the subway, get off at Park Avenue station in Manhattan, and go to the street level to look for the street number. We can make it. We're familiar with a subway system, not this kind, but still a subway. Let's go to bed; otherwise, we will be late tomorrow."

"Alex, you know I don't drink, but I wish I had something to celebrate."

"Are you sure?" Alex asked and pulled a small bottle of whisky from the luggage.

They laughed, had a sip, and fell asleep happy.

* * * *

The time was so different in America; they would need a few days just to get used to the new time. Ana hadn't slept well, thinking about the meeting, scared of being late.

She prepared everything Sarah would need to get dressed, as much as she could, without her mom's help. Then, she put together Phillip's outfit and felt grateful his clothes looked ok, because she had forgotten to pull them from the suitcase when they arrived the night before.

She told Sarah that they would have to leave her alone because of the meeting and that Phillip would go with them.

Sarah wanted to make her mom's life easier and said, "You know I will be here, waiting for you. I won't go anywhere."

Alex, Ana, and Phillip went to the subway station and changed the money they had to get quarters to pay for the ride. Ana put the quarters in the special box, asked Phillip to go under the bar, and she followed him. Alex used another entrance so they could be ready at the same time.

Suddenly, a loud whistle filled the whole space, making everybody look back towards the cashier's cabin. Ana continued walking, holding Phillip's hand, knowing she did everything she had to do. Somebody tapped her on her shoulder and asked her to go back to the cashier's cabin. Ana went back there.

Alex was waiting for her, wondering what went wrong.

Phillip was shaking, scared and wanting to be with his mom. He was afraid somebody would hurt her.

Ana looked at the person that stopped her and said, "Do you want to talk to me? I think it is a mistake."

"No, it is not a mistake, it is you."

"Why?"

"You pushed your child under the bar without paying money for him. There is a stick located on the right side of the gate. If the child is taller than the stick, you have to pay the same amount that you paid for you. Your son is taller than the stick and you have to put money in the machine."

"But he is only eight years old!"

"Doesn't matter the age, it's about how tall he is. That's the rule."

Ana put money in the designated space and they finally got into the subway wagon. She just learned her first lesson, and she knew many other lessons would come. They were so afraid of being late for their meeting. Anybody could easily guess they were foreigners. The way they were dressed and the way they looked around.

At least the address wasn't hard to find.

The building was elegant and in an old style. They had to take the elevator all the way to the twelfth floor. What magnificence! The inside of the building had a very impressive lobby, very elegant. Ana and her family were so nervous about the meeting.

After waiting a few minutes, a nice lady wearing heavy glasses came and introduced herself, "Hi, my name is Ms. Meredith and I will be your caseworker. I will take care of your family. Welcome to America, we are glad to have you here. We need people like you. Where is the fourth member of your family?"

"Hi, Ms. Meredith, our daughter is wheelchair-bound and she stayed home."

"Oh, of course, you had no transportation set up for her yet. Don't worry. Soon, she will be able to go everywhere. That's why I am here, to help you get situated." She invited them into her office and read all their folders again, to be sure she wasn't missing something important. She said, "It will take a little bit longer than other cases, but it will be done right and as fast as I can. Mr. Phillip," she said, looking at Ana's son, "Sir, you are already a very handsome young man. You're going to get all the required immunizations at this location." She circled an address on a document full of addresses that she gave to his mother.

Phillip's eyes were wide open, smiling because he didn't

understand one word from what the lady said.

His mom whispered in his ears that she would explain later what she'd said.

Ms. Meredith continued, "Once he's done with the immunizations, you have to register him at this school." She circled another address. "So, Mr. Phillip…for some reason, I like to call him like that; it sounds so nice, will start school right away. He will be the first one to be integrated into the system." Ms. Meredith hugged Phillip.

This made Ana feel so good, so welcomed and everybody was smiling.

"Ok, now let's move to another folder. Mr. Alex, I will make arrangements for you to go and learn English as a second language. There are churches offering classes. I will find one closer to your apartment. Are you ok with this? If you find somewhere to work, you are free to do so because you have a green card and the right to work. Paying taxes for what you earn. But the most important thing is the language. I noticed you know some, but it has to be better."

"Yes, ma'am, I will get better. I cannot wait to start it."

"Ana, now it is your turn. I am so glad you speak English. I will set up some appointments for you to have job interviews. I see in your folder that you have two main qualifications: blueprint technician for chemical industry and the cosmetic field. I would suggest trying the industrial jobs first. This way, the salary will be higher and you can have better benefits: retirement, 401(k), and a lot more. What do you think about that?"

"I will be so happy to get a job as soon as possible. Thank you." Ana felt confused though. What is a 401(k)? What does 'benefits' mean? But she kept listening, polite and quiet.

"Ok. Now…Sarah's situation. How is her health? I will do my best for your daughter, to get everything she might need to become an independent person, to go to school and maybe later on, get a job. Once she starts using transportation, we'll make an appointment here, so I can meet her."

"Ok, I will bring her here. When will her appointment be? And she loves school. Sarah loves to study; she will be an excellent student."

"I will connect you with a transportation company that will take her to school and to her medical appointments. You have to take her to a Social Security office, to get her Medicaid card." Ms. Meredith realized they had no idea about all the terms she used, and she said she would explain everything when the time came. She knew it was a lot of information to digest. "Mr. Alex, this is a book of food stamps; there are coupons for one month."

Ana and Alex had never heard about "food stamps," but they realized it was something connected with food. Ana's mind went back to her country when she heard about coupons; she wondered how it was possible to get food using coupons, here in the USA? She knew later on she would understand the system, but now she was so confused.

Thank God, Ms. Meredith continued to explain, "When you go to the grocery store, select the food you need. Once you've finished, give the coupon book to the cashier and she will cut as many as needed to cover the food cost. Then, she will give the rest back to you. But be aware, not all items are covered by food stamps, like paper towels, toilet paper, hot or prepared food, alcohol, and a lot more. You will learn as you go. And you are going to get a small amount of money to help you get started. Let's make another appointment so we can discuss your progress and anything else that needs to be done to get you going. I'm sure you will achieve great success; something tells me. I like being your caseworker already." She hugged them, and they could feel how sincere she was.

"Alex, we have a good start. Ms. Meredith is a good woman, and she will take good care of us; I know it."

They left the building, wandering around a bit, but in a hurry to get back to Sarah. Their daughter was so happy to see them back; not that she had been scared, not because she was alone, but because she knew her family was in a huge, unknown city. The superintendent checked on her to be sure she was ok. He was an unbelievably good man. Ana told him that they had to be in Manhattan at a certain time for an interview, but he was used to such things. Ana's family wasn't the first one to be hosted in his building.

He called the building 'his building,' because he got to know everybody and he had to fix everything that was broken, day or night.

* * * *

The next morning, Ana took Phillip to get his immunizations so he could start school. Alex stayed home with Sarah. Somebody knocked at their door, it was the superintendent.

"Alex, if you have time, let's go in the basement and you can choose things that you need for your family. You will need metal frames for your mattresses, some tables, a microwave, dishes, blinds, curtains, and whatever you think you might need. Is your wife home? Because she knows what she needs for her family, and you can get the man stuff, tools and who knows what else. You wouldn't believe how many things are there!"

"Come inside, please. Let me get ready to go with you. I have to leave things for Sarah that she can grab and show her how the TV works."

"Ok, take your time. I'll have a chance to talk to your daughter. My wife is pregnant and soon, we're going to have a baby boy."

"Congratulations, you will be the best father in the world."

"I think you are not too bad, either."

It seemed they liked each other and you could sense the good vibes coming from this man. He had compassion for their family; he could imagine how hard it was to raise a child in a wheelchair and to come from a foreign country starting from scratch. He had a deep admiration for them, and it was reflected in his eyes and actions. Nobody asked him to knock at the door and offer help. God was working already—actually, he never stopped.

When Ana and Phillip came back from the clinic, they couldn't believe the changes in their apartment. Sarah's eyes were so happy, looking around her and seeing how things were coming together. Soon, the beds were ready with sheets, pillows, and blankets; the dishes they needed were in the cabinets, and it seemed like a magic wand worked above them all. The family had never lived in such a large apartment.

Phillip started school and his mother knew it would be hard for the first two or three months, until he started speaking English.

"Hi, my son, how was your day at school?" From now on, she would only ask him in English, she promised herself.

"Everybody was so nice with me, but I have no idea what they said. They gave me pens and a notebook; and I already learned to count in English. I like this language."

"Soon, you will speak English like your classmates."

"I want to, so I can play games with them. The teacher is very nice and she let me use my left hand. This makes me happy. Mom, you know almost everybody in my class has dark colored skin; why do they have dark skin?"

"Phillip, not all people have your coloring. Some are white, some dark, some yellow. We are all different, but the same. You and I never saw a dark skinned person, only in the movies, but now we're going to live together, and they will be your friends and mine."

"Ok, I understand. I was just curious why they have a different color than I do."

"Good, so tomorrow you will play with everybody like you did in Bucharest."

"I did play today, too."

Sarah started using the provided transportation to go to her new school. The bus provided a ramp so she could go with her wheelchair. Her school was in Manhattan, and she couldn't be more pleased to attend such a school. She already knew some English, but she had to perfect it. She loved English so much, that this was the least of Ana's problems. She knew how much her daughter wanted to go to school, because she'd never had this opportunity.

Alex was going to his English classes and making good progress. The family started communicating only in English, to expedite the learning process, plus they enjoyed it.

Ana had a notebook full of addresses for a variety of job interviews. She made the appointments and presented herself with dignity and knowledge.

"Ana, you are an excellent technician, but you're used to the

European measurement system, and we use the American one. They are so different. It will take time for you to learn our system. Give us a call when you get American experience. We will hire you right away."

Ana felt so confused, and she couldn't understand why she was sent to those interviews if the caseworker knew she might not be accepted. Ana was the only one right now who could go to work and bring money home, and she wasn't able to find a job. She decided to call her sponsor and tell her everything she was going through. "Ms. Meredith, may I come and talk to you? I am sorry to bother you, but I need your help."

"Hi, Ana, I have an opening today at three o'clock. Can you come?"

"Thank you, I will be there. Thank you."

Ana made arrangements for Sarah to find everything she needed until Alex came home, and she took the subway to meet her caseworker.

"Hi, Ana, what's happened; what's wrong? You are so pale!"

"Hi, Ms. Meredith, am I? I know I am because I'm very upset. Every day I spent money on the subway, going from one interview to another. All the answers are the same: come back once you have the American experience. How can I get this if nobody accepts me, to give me chance to show what I can do, to show them what I know? Ms. Meredith, please, tell me where to go, what to do. I have to find a job."

"Didn't you have other skills? I remembered you have something with cosmetics, am I right?"

"Yes, you are, but you said I would be much better off getting a job in my primary field and that's why you gave me all those addresses."

"I remember, but maybe we have to switch the plan. Let me think about it and give me a call in a few days. Ana, everything will be just fine. Look at your family. Everybody has a schedule; they go to schools and they're happy. But it seems that you want things done yesterday. Be patient; you have what you need to have a decent life."

"Thank you, Ms. Meredith. I needed to talk to you. I feel much better now; thank you. I will call you in two days."

Ms. Meredith knew that Ana was different from most of the women she helped. When Ana said she would call in two days, she realized that Ana had set up her own time, not the caseworker. Ms. Meredith said, "Call me in a few days," not two days! She realized this woman would be a very successful one; she was so determined to work, to make a living. What a woman!

* * * *

Ana left the office feeling much lighter, full of hope that she would find a job soon. She was smiling and suddenly remembered one of the first things her caseworker told all of them… "No eye contact." It was almost impossible for all of them to understand the meaning of her advice. They were used to smiling at people, to holding doors for those that needed it, being friendly. How could somebody ask such a stupid thing? They talked about it, but they weren't able to find a solution, until now.

"Beautiful lady, how are you? You seem to be so lonely. What about a drink?" somebody said to Ana, getting closer to her. She sensed the danger and was wondering why this man talked to her that way. *Oh, now I know. I was smiling like a stupid woman, looking to find something for her —My God, I am so stupid. Ms. Meredith told us from the first day, do not look around like we don't know where we are and don't make eye contact, and here I am smiling at everybody.* She walked faster and rushed to the subway station, grateful that the guy didn't follow her.

When she got home, she told Alex what happened and she promised to be more careful when she was alone.

There was a small grocery store close to their building and they decided to go there and buy food. Everybody got dressed like they were going to a theater or for a nice visit. They had the beautiful clothes from the Jewish Federation. Ana pushed the shopping cart and Alex pushed Sarah's wheelchair. Phillip wandered around the shelves, touching and smelling everything he could reach, and said, "Mom, look at this; look at that! Mom, I want them all." He grabbed what he liked and put them in the shopping cart.

"Son, come closer, please, and listen to what I am telling you now. First, I want you to look at the price label and if the price is over one dollar, you put it back."

"Why? I want them."

"We cannot afford to buy things like this now, but I promise you we will. For now, just what is necessary. Extra things later on, not now. Thank you, son, for understanding. I love you." Ana was surprised to see Phillip grabbing the sweets and putting them back on the shelves. "Thank you son, the day will come and you can buy things more expensive than one dollar."

When the family approached the cashier, Ana looked around because she sensed something. She noticed people behind them were talking about her family! Ana was holding the food stamp coupons like a checkbook, it was wide open and could be seen by everybody around and behind her. Even if she knew she shouldn't smile, she did anyway.

Nobody smiled back to her. She knew something was going on. She noticed that her family was dressed a lot different than people in the grocery store. She had high heels and an elegant outfit. Alex was wearing a long-sleeve, quality shirt. Phillip had a brand- new jacket and colorful sneakers. Sarah was all put together and her clothes had coordinated colors.

Overall, they looked like they could pay with "real" money, not food stamps. Ana could feel their thoughts, and she didn't blame them for being hostile. People were judging them by their appearance. These people had no idea where the clothes came from, what Ana and her family had to endure to be where they were now. These people had no idea they just arrived in this country and were looking for jobs.

Another lesson was learned that day. After she "paid" for the food, she grabbed her family and left the store in a hurry. Nobody could understand why she was in such a hurry.

"Alex, today was the last day I will use the food stamps. I have to find a job as soon as possible to make money."

"But you are going for job interviews every day. What's

happened that you look so stressed out? You look like you are ready
to cry."

"I am." She told them what she just went through, and they all
decided to wear not-so-nice clothes until they found jobs.

* * * *

Ana told her caseworker about the grocery store incident and
asked her to accelerate the job-finding process, if she could.

"Ana, you have to understand that it's not a shame to use those
food stamps. There are situations in life when somebody has to use
them. But I admire your tenacity and persistence to get a job. Do
you know something? What about going for a job interview at a
famous salon on Madison Avenue in Manhattan? The manager of
the salon is a Russian lady that was our client, like you are now.
Let's change the field, maybe there are more jobs in the cosmetic
field than the blueprints."

"Ms. Meredith, I will do everything you tell me to do."

Ana's caseworker arranged for her to test her skills, and she
hoped the manager of the skin-care salon would offer her a job.

Ana was nervous this time. She was a lot more confident in the
blueprint drawing field than skin care. She hadn't practiced her
passion for skin care in a long time. The only thing she knew was
that she would really love to work on clients, to make them happy.
But she knew she wasn't ready to get such a job.

She purchased a white top, looking like a uniform, in order to
improve her appearance for the job, to look like an aesthetician. She
arrived early for her appointment, and the manager greeted her and
invited her to one of their treatment rooms. A model, a "guinea pig,"
was waiting for Ana to work on her skin. The only thing the manager
wanted to see was the face massage, to see Ana's technique and how
she approached the "client." Ana washed her hands and started
massaging the model's face, neck, and décolleté.

The manager called a few of the aestheticians that were
available and asked them to watch Ana's hands.

This made Ana even more nervous, but she finished the

massage, then thanked the model for offering to be her guinea pig.

The model was an aesthetician working there and she thanked Ana for making her feel really good.

The manager thanked Ana and told her to come back as soon as she got her license, and she promised her she would have a job at their salon.

Ana was "flying" more than walking. She was so happy. She went directly to her caseworker to tell her the good news.

"So, what did she say?"

"It seemed like she liked my technique and she offered me a job, once I get my license. What is this, a license?"

"Oh, no! It is exactly what I was afraid of. You know, Ana. I wasn't sure how things worked in this specific field, and I thought she would offer you a job there, a regular job, not as an aesthetician. I hoped they could offer a 'learning on the spot' program, and this way you could get your license later on. A license is an authorization obtained after a state board exam that allows you to perform services for clients."

"Oh, how do I get this paper? How much does it cost?"

"Ana, it is not that simple. In order to be admitted to take the board exam, you have to graduate a specific school, to get a few thousand hours of training and education. It is a long process, and it is the only one to get your license. Let me see how we can do this for you, because the schooling takes a few months and you need to make money working." She thought for a moment and continued, "Maybe we can find an evening school. This way, you can go to work during the day and to school in the evenings. Ana, something will come up, for sure. Cosmetics or blueprint, you'll see." She hugged Ana, feeling sorry that she couldn't help her like she helped so many hundreds of clients. Ana's family was so different; their needs were harder to meet, but as a caseworker, she had to fight for them, to help them to get jobs so they could live on their own.

"Ms. Meredith, thank you for your hard work, but I cannot go to an evening school when my son is only eight years old. Alex is helping our superintendent to paint some apartments in our building so we can get some money. Sarah needs help in the house when she comes back from school. I have to find something, but as soon as you send me somewhere for job interviews, I will go right away."

Ana went home determined to get a job, any job! Their building was located on a central avenue in Brooklyn, separating two distinct contrasts, the very rich Jewish area with mansions and twenty-four-hour police patrol, cameras, and no subway access. The other side was crowded by poor buildings, old apartment buildings, unsafe streets, and dangerous places to raise a family, to let your children out. Ana was shocked to find out about the "Jewish" community. She was wondering if she had something in common with the Jewish people, asking herself why, everywhere she lived, it seemed to be close to the Jewish people. But this time, her fate had nothing to do with the Jewish community, even if she wished for the opposite, to get help again.

* * * *

Ana had some free time; the children were in school and Alex was working with the superintendent of their building. She noticed there were a few businesses located on their avenue. One of them was a hair salon. She went directly there. When she opened the door, she realized absolutely everybody was African American. They looked like really nice ladies, and they smiled when she greeted them. At least, she felt at ease.

The owner of the salon looked at her from head to toes and asked, "Are you looking for a haircut?"

"Oh no, ma'am, I am looking for a job."

"Did you ever shampoo our type of hair?"

"No, never, but if you show me how to do it, I will be more than happy to do it. I am new to this country. I am legal here. And I have to make some money till I get a real job."

"Where do you live?"

Ana told the owner where her apartment was.

The owner seemed to like it being so close, so Ana wouldn't be late to work. "Ok," she said. "Just watch me how I do it."

Ana paid close attention to everything the lady was doing,

learning really fast. The first shampoos were hard to do because of the difference in the hair texture. It was so much different than her hair, or her family's hair, but she learned how to manage it.

She showed up every day that she wasn't going to job interviews. The clients of that salon started to like the way she was massaging their scalp, neck, and shoulders when they were waiting for the hairstylist. They asked for her when they made their appointments. The owner was very happy to work less, and Ana was extremely happy with the tips from the clients. The owner was paying her a few dollars per hour, but the tips helped a lot with the family expenses.

Ana was able to keep her promise…she never used the food stamps again. The family had a lot less money than if they would have kept using the food stamps, but they were a lot happier to feel free to buy food like any other American person. Ana didn't need a license to do what she was doing at the salon, but she knew she had to obtain that paper to get a better job. Actually, she was never technically hired at the salon; she was only helping the owner.

When the clients were waiting with the color on their hair, Ana would exfoliate and massage their faces, applying masks she made especially for them. She brought all the ingredients from her apartment and she "cooked" them in front of the client. People spread the word about how good and different Ana was, so they started requesting skin treatments with her. The only problem was that she couldn't perform those services because she didn't have the special license needed for that kind of service.

CHAPTER FOURTEEN

Sarah came home from school and couldn't stop saying how much better her life was since she came to America, thanking their parents for bringing her to this country. "Mom, I cannot believe it. There are ramps everywhere, handrails, bathrooms with special signs and large enough to turn a wheelchair! It's so easy to go everywhere you want. God bless this country. I have friends now, and my teachers love me. My English is getting so much better that I can write essays and write papers for my courses."

"I'm so happy for you and for us. Our dreams will become reality soon. Look at your brother; he speaks English like all the kids in his class. No accent. He's lost his Romanian accent and lately, he answers in English when we ask something. I want him to keep speaking the Romanian language. It will be a good brain exercise for him, to make his brain translate. But lately, he prefers only English."

"Mom, he will speak only English. Look at me, I already prefer English; it comes easily for me."

"I am so proud of you both. Actually, I'm proud of your father too. His English is getting so much clearer, and the fact that he works with the super—it helps him a lot because he has to communicate in English. It is me that needs help, and I am going to find something soon. It has been almost four months since we came here."

In the days after her conversation with her daughter, Ana felt like God was telling her something. Things in the apartment were in order, the food ready, the children were in school, and Alex was working with the super. The same scenario as the day she entered the hair salon. This time, she tried something different. She got dressed in one of the beautiful outfits she brought from her country, wearing decent heels, light makeup, and nice earrings.

Ana took the subway all the way to Fifth Avenue, the spine of Manhattan. Her intuition was telling her that Manhattan was the answer to her prayers. When she got out to the street level, she tried to look like a local not like a visitor, and she remembered the first advice she got from her caseworker, Ms. Meredith…no eye contact, no smiling. The first building that impressed her was Macy's. She knew the name from the commercials and knew it was a high-quality department store.

"Ok, let me go inside and see what it is all about." The moment she entered the store, an amazing fragrance covered her like a blanket, reminding her of the duty-free shop from Bucharest, where her friend worked. The French fragrance…

She could spend hours here, looking, touching, and smelling all the good stuff. Ana wanted the day to never end. She wanted to stay there and forget about everything. She wanted to work here, to find a job, any job, just to work there. So, Ana walked around the store for several minutes. She was attracted by a name that she'd known for many years, a French company. She approached the salesperson. "Hi, may I talk to the manager, please?"

"Do you have an appointment?"

"No, but I would like to talk to her, if it is possible."

The salesperson must have like Ana because she went behind the counter and talked to her manager in her office. When she came back, she told Ana, "You are lucky. She will be here shortly."

"Thank you so much, I appreciate what you did." Ana's face and thoughts radiated happiness. It is a beginning. Somebody will talk to me. I can do any kind of job here, whatever they need. I will do it."

A tiny lady came and introduced herself. She looked at Ana from head to toe, like the other lady from the hair salon in her neighborhood did. Hopefully, this was be a good sign.

"Thank you for taking the time to talk to me. I was wondering what kind of spa treatments you offer here."

The manager invited Ana to follow her and she opened the door of a treatment room. Ana looked at the equipment and said, "I see that you use two machines; I used five!"

"Ok, let's talk."

Ana had studied cosmetic techniques, procedures and skin care ingredients with a French trainer, back when she was a lot younger. But it had been Ana's mother who instilled her love for beauty, a love for respecting her skin and she taught her as much as she knew. She remembered how women were taking care of their skin even if they had no money for food. It was like a cult, all of them trying to look good, clean and have good skin. Whatever you were eating: fruits, vegetables, eggs, cucumbers, honey, milk, were going on your face too! Her mother loved beauty, and she kept pushing it on her daughters. She never thought that her "hobby" would become her real profession. But it did; Ana got the job and was hired by a reputable cosmetics company.

When Ana was in training, she used many pieces of equipment she never thought she would ever use again. Her job was secure, and she had enjoyed the blueprint drawing, even while she'd considered the aesthetics secondary. All the way home, she couldn't stop thanking God for the gift she'd just received, her job! The subway was running too slow for Ana; she wanted to get home fast and tell everybody how happy she was.

The job would give Ana and her family good benefits, health insurance, and a good salary. She had to be in training for a full month, and she had to be under the supervision of a master cosmetologist for a certain amount of time in order to take the board exam. It couldn't get better than this.

* * * *

Ana missed Sophia, who lived far away from her, and was happy when she came to visit the family, to see how they settled in, how were they doing.

They would talk on the phone every day, mostly about the family. Sophia's love for animals was making her an advocate for animal rights. She adopted a few cats and dogs, even if she knew this "love" would cost money. Sophia spent a fortune on her "children" and her wardrobe; she loved luxury.

Ana realized that how Sophia acted was a consequence of the way her father raised her, giving her everything she wanted. Of course, at his financial level, she was used to the good stuff.

"I'm so glad you are here in America. It will be so much easier for Sarah to live here, to become independent. I can tell already, by looking at her, how much better she is. And Phillip is absolutely the most handsome young man I ever saw."

"Of course, he's your nephew! You see him with different eyes. I know you're right though. I look at him and thank God for such a gift. The first thing he noticed and was happy about was that the teacher let him write with his left hand. He was happy. His English is almost perfect. The kids learned fast and they don't have the accent like we do. Look at you, being so young, you have no accent and your English is so beautiful."

"I'm so happy you got that job. I am ok with mine. I do what I studied for, but for me to become a complete engineer, I have to take the board—a very long, difficult exam in order to get the 'stamp.'"

"Food stamps? I'm kidding. I understand. I will have to pass the cosmetology board exam to become a cosmetologist and be allowed to do all the services listed on my job description. Now I can only do them if my supervisor is there. Sophia, I got to meet famous movie stars, politicians that I only read about in the magazines. I was nervous in the beginning, but now I am very comfortable working on them."

They had a good time together and talked a lot about their relatives. The love they both had for their cousins and all the people they left there—it made them sad, but at the same time, sharing memories made them laugh and enjoy each second spent together.

Time went by too quickly and Sophia had to go back to her husband and her animals. She felt good seeing her sister and spending some time together. So many memories. Both sisters made plans to bring their mom for a visit. She was getting older, and she would need her daughters.

Escape

* * * *

Ana was very much appreciated at work. She'd taken the exam and passed it with high grades. Alex was saving all the money he was getting from working with the super, and soon, they purchased a van to take Sarah places and for all of them to go out of the city, when they could. This made Ana think about what her manager had told everybody yesterday, "Ok, see you all Monday!"

Ana remembered being confused at the announcement. "Oh, wait a minute, please, why Monday? I can be here tomorrow."

"Ana tomorrow is Saturday, and we have two days off. Enjoy your family and your days off."

"Ok, but I want to work. I need the money."

"It is part of your monthly salary. So, have a nice weekend. Get some rest too."

"Ok, thank you. See you Monday."

Ana had been sad and happy at the same time. She needed to learn how the system worked. When she got home, she prepared things for the next day. "Let's see what a day off can do for us!"

"Guys, today and tomorrow we can do whatever you want!"

"Are you sure? It is Saturday and you go to work."

"No, I have two days off."

"Did they fire you?"

"Not yet!" she answered, smiling.

Alex was so happy to be able to take his family to beautiful places, there were so many; so much to learn, to explore, to get to know their city.

Long Island was their favorite place to go. Alex and Phillip would play tennis, while Ana and Sarah would visit the surroundings, the park and many stores. The place had a special charm for them.

* * * *

"So, how was your weekend?" Ana's manager asked.

"Very good. Thank you so much for asking. I think it will not be hard to get used to the good things."

"I'm glad you enjoyed it." She thought for a moment and continued, "Ana, I will always remember the day I handed you your first paycheck; I will never forget your eyes. You opened the envelope and asked, 'Where is the money?' And I told you that that check represented your money, your payment."

"Then I asked you, 'What am I supposed to do with this paper?'"

"So, did you go to the bank? Did somebody there help you open an account and deposit the check? And were you given a few temporary checks after someone showed you what to do with the checks, how to make payments for your bills?"

"Yes, all is ok, and now I understand. In my country, the salary was always cash. They would take out whatever you owe to the government and give you the rest. We never had checks, but I will learn it. Thank you."

"By the way, do you remember the movie star you worked on last week?"

"Yes, I do. She was a very nice lady."

"Well, she booked her next appointment and asked for you. What a compliment! Ana, you will be our star soon."

One day, after Ana finished the treatment for a client, she received a business card with a nice tip. She was in a hurry to clean her room and get it ready for the next client.

She put the business card in her pocket and forgot about it. When she got on the bus to go home, she grabbed the card from her pocket and read it. It was the client's name and underneath was, *"Headhunter!"* Ana thought she hadn't read it right. "What does a headhunter have to do with me; why did she give me her card?" She almost ignored it, but the next morning, she decided to show it to a coworker.

Her friend looked at the business card and said, "Lucky you!"

"What do you mean lucky me? I don't hunt."

"Ana, a headhunter offers you a job; it is a person looking for quality workers for different companies. They send her to get services done, our type of services, and if she is impressed with the technician, she leaves her business card. People know about this. She wants to offer you a much better job with more money, for sure."

"Oh, thank you for teaching me all those new things. I'm very happy here and I love what I do. It feels good to see that you are appreciated." She went back to doing what she liked the most, beauty treatments. So much elegance, the nice people, the fragrances. Ana never dreamed she would work in such a place. Blessings were pouring from the sky. She couldn't be more grateful.

* * * *

Ms. Meredith couldn't believe how fast Ana and the entire family had adjusted, how fast they were able to give up the "government help." No more food stamps, no more money to pay the bills. And all this in less than half of the year! It was a record, considering how difficult their case was. Ms. Meredith was using them as an example for everybody. If this family with two children, one wheelchair-bound, was able to do it, anybody could do it.

But at the same time, she knew that Ana and Alex were made of different stuff. They'd suffered under the Communist regime; they had to survive with almost nothing. Her admiration went beyond work boundaries; she asked them to keep in touch and be friends. Normally, Ms. Meredith wasn't allowed to keep a friendship with her clients, but she had so much respect for Ana's family that she had to ask them to remain friends, and they did.

* * * *

Alex's English was getting so good that he felt he could go to college to become a physical therapist. The college he graduated from in Bucharest had the physical therapy credits incorporated in his degree. So, Alex went to Hunter College in Manhattan to check into how those credits might apply.

Otherwise, life seemed to be coming together for all of them. Phillip was the happiest to spend time with his father. He adored

Alex, and their time together was priceless. The memories they created would last a lifetime; each second spent together was precious.

Ana was always working and had to do so many other things in the apartment, so she couldn't spend as much time with Phillip as Alex did. She knew it; she could see and feel the difference between the love her son had for his father and the love he had for her. This made her sad and "jealous," but in a good way. She always thought that a mother's job was to be home when her kids came home from school. But it is one thing to know it, and one thing to be able to do it. She had to work; she loved to work.

She had to bring money home and she hoped it wouldn't leave deep marks between her son and her. She loved him more than anybody could comprehend.

Phillip was her soul, her gift from God; he was the reason they had a family. He was the reason Sarah wasn't alone. He gave life back to his parents. Phillip was the glue for his family.

Ana had tears in her eyes every time she looked at her son. He was smart, very well built for his age, and he enjoyed playing sports so much with his father. Her tears were tears of happiness, tears of love.

When she'd given birth to Phillip, God renewed her lease on happiness.

Ana hoped things would change, so she would be able to spend more time with her son and be home when he would come back from school.

* * * *

One day, Ana came home and prepared dinner for her family. When they finished eating, she announced, "I have some good news for us. I will go to Paris, and you can join me," she said, looking at Alex. "The plane tickets will be paid for by my company. They love me so much."

"Are you talking about me? Oh, no. I am not going anywhere. It isn't ok to make them pay for me. I don't work there. And on top of everything, who will take care of Phillip? I won't leave him here without us. I don't trust somebody to take care of him, to take him to school and bring him back."

"No, the company will pay for the hotel room and for a babysitter."

"What? Are they insane? It will cost lots of money. I know how much they appreciate you, but I never thought they could spend so much money. You go, and I will stay here and take care of Phillip and Sarah."

"Sarah is ok. She can do so much now."

However, Ana went to Paris alone and even still, it was one the most beautiful presents of her life. Before she came back from Paris, the host invited her to spend France's Independence Day on a boat along the river, eating dinner, drinking wine, and listening to music. What a night; what a joy! She missed her family and she promised herself that one day, they would spend a vacation in Paris, the City of Lights. Her knowledge of skin care, her techniques, and her approach toward clients was a gift she offered to her French colleagues. Ana came back home and her family greeted her with love. She could see how much she was missed.

"Did you miss me because of what I do for you, or because you just missed me for me?"

"Mom, I missed you very much. Don't go again; stay home with me," Phillip insisted.

"Ok, son, I will. I love you so much. I missed you a lot it's good to be home. Alex, we have to spend a vacation there; it is absolutely fantastic."

"Maybe, one day…it would be nice."

Ana went back to work the next day and everything seemed to go back to normal.

* * * *

Sarah's physical condition remained the same and Ana knew that her daughter's diagnosis was a permanent one, but she was impressed to see how many things she could do on her own. Now

Sarah could get around by herself. She had freedom—a new, completely different life, and a much better life. Sarah had never dreamed of being independent; she never thought this could happen to her.

"Now I understand what it means to be independent. I still need help, but I can do so much more. This powered wheelchair is my independence, Mom. I'm so happy! Do you have few minutes for me? I need to talk to you."

"I always have a few minutes for you, since you were born. Give me a few minutes to finish this thing."

"I know you always have time for me, but this is different."

"Ok, let's talk, my sweet baby."

"I'm not a baby anymore and I have met somebody."

"What? What did you just say? I am so happy for you. Go ahead. Tell me, I'm so anxious to hear about him."

"He's a very nice man and I like him."

"That's all? Tell me more, more, please."

They giggled to each other.

"I met him at school."

"Is he in a wheelchair too?"

"No, he walks like everybody else, but I think he has something else, like lupus. I know it is an immune system disease. I read about it because I want to help him as much as I can."

"I'm sorry for him, but in this country, there are so many chances he will find a solution for his condition."

"Is it ok to go and see a movie with him tomorrow?"

"Do you even need to ask? Of course, bring him over after the movie."

"I will, but what about Papa? You know how he is."

"Don't worry about him. I will take care of this. I will cook some pasta; what do you think?"

"Perfect, he is Italian!"

Both of them had a good laugh, and anyone could see how happy they were, how much they loved each other, mother and daughter.

Ana prayed that Sarah would know what love was all about.

Sarah had so much to offer and Ana hoped people would see her first, not her wheelchair. When she was younger, she used to write poems. The way she put the words together, her imagination reflected a different way of seeing her surroundings. A flower was just a flower for most people but for her, that flower could symbolize, represent something else, that flower could have a meaning and a purpose, could have healing properties, the fragrance, the color, the petals. She was very quiet but very busy inside; this was Sarah. You needed time to get to know her.

* * * *

"Alex, our daughter has a boyfriend."

"What does 'a boyfriend' mean? A real boyfriend, you say?"

"Well, I'm not sure yet. I know we are old fashioned parents, but we live in a free country with different conceptions, different standards."

"No, the standards are the same. But I will wait to meet him and then we'll talk again. I want to be sure she is safe, first of all."

Sarah came home after the movie and introduced her boyfriend to her family.

Phillip was all ready to inspect him worse than the FBI. He checked him head to toe and got closer to his sister, ready to protect her. Ana pulled him towards her, so the poor guy wouldn't feel uncomfortable.

"This is Edmond," Sarah said, smiling.

"What kind of name is that?" Phillip asked.

"Italian, I'm Italian. What is your name?"

"Phillip, nice to meet you."

Ana noticed that her husband didn't look too happy, but he was polite. "Let's have dinner."

She invited everybody to sit down and enjoy her cooking. She wanted to know Edmond better; to be sure her daughter was in good hands. She was afraid they would have no conversation going on because they didn't know each other, but thank God, Edmond was very talkative, enough to save the evening. Ana knew that her husband wouldn't like how much Edmond talked, but she was grateful somebody was talking.

Sarah enjoyed listening to him, and this was great. Sarah being quiet, it was good for her to have somebody like Edmond entertaining her.

Phillip had a chance to practice his English, and he had fun learning a few new things from Edmond. He almost liked him.

Ana invited Edmond to come back every time he took Sarah out to spend some time together.

Not too long after that dinner, Sarah came home from school and asked her parents if she could move out and live with Edmond, in his apartment!

Now, the volcano erupted! Ana's mind was a volcano and heard this conversation going on in her mind: *No, absolutely not! You are not married to him; you cannot live together. First, you have to get married, then you move out. How do you dare to even ask such a thing?* But she kept it to herself, wanting to talk to Alex first.

Both of them were so upset that they couldn't sleep the whole night. Different scenarios were moving in their minds with Sarah in different situations, wondering how she was going to do things, who was going to help her, and a lot of other questions connected to her physical disability.

In the morning, Ana asked her daughter, "Sarah, where are you going to live? Who's going to help you, like I do?"

"Edmond. He lives in an apartment, but the building is an old one and doesn't have wheelchair accessibility. He will help me to do things. He said he is going to put my name on a waiting list through Catholic Charities to get a studio on my own and we can move together. This organization has buildings equipped with everything for elderly and disabled people, so they can live there doing things on their own. All my life, I have heard: 'I want you to be independent, to be able to live on your own once your father and me will be gone from this world,' am I right?"

"Yes, you are. But as a mother, I can tell that you like Edmond, but you don't love him. Sarah, it is a huge difference between liking somebody and loving somebody. Time will tell, unfortunately. But he is a nice man, and he is in love with you, this I can tell."

"Mother, you're right. I don't need time to tell, but he makes me feel loved, beautiful, and appreciated as a woman. I feel the same way with you, but you are my parents. He's a man and he loves me. Will I marry him? I'm not sure right now. He wants to, but I have other things in my mind."

Alex was listening and he didn't say one word, but he knew his baby girl was right. She was a grown-up young woman now. She had to meet the world. It was her time now. "Ana, we have to let her move out. I never thought I would say these words."

"I think so, too. Let her life begin."

It didn't take long for Sarah to move to Edmond's apartment. Ana invited them to spend the weekend, to have a nice time as a family. Phillip was the happiest. "Yes, let's get together," he said. "I miss Sarah. Our apartment is so quiet now, without her."

"What do you mean? She didn't talk much anyway. She was very quiet."

"Yes, but not with me," Phillip answered.

Ana looked at Alex and they agreed that Phillip was right. When Sarah and Edmond arrived, the apartment was full of life again. What a difference one loved person could make! They were playing games, laughing and clearly happy to be with each other.

Ana watched Sarah, making sure she was doing well, that she was truly happy with Edmond.

Phillip didn't want Sarah to leave their apartment again; he was glued to her. The time came to say goodbye and Phillip looked ready to cry.

Ana put her arm around him so he could feel her love.

Sarah promised to come more often to spend more time with her loved ones. "Mom, thank you for everything you do for me, and Edmond, too. We have the best food in the building. You save us so much money, thank you. I will become lazy if you keep cooking for us."

"I do it with love. I'm happy to see you doing well and to see how much this man loves you. It makes us, me and your father, worry less."

A few days after having "the children" in their apartment for the weekend, Sarah called her mother and was so happy she could barely talk. "Mom, my name came up on the list and soon, I'm going to receive my own studio, my own. Handicap access—with everything I need to live on my own! Mom, I am so happy. We have to celebrate; this is a huge gift for my life. There will be so many things to take care of. I will have a lease and I have to pay utilities, the phone; and I will be responsible for all these things, like any other person! This is a privilege. I am my own boss."

"Sarah," Ana started, wondering if she had finished talking, "I am so excited for the good news, but I worry now. Who's going to help you shower, cook, dress, and so many other things? Is Edmond going to move with you?"

"He can, but I told him that if something happened between us, and we didn't get along anymore, he would have no place to go. Once he gives up his apartment, somebody else from the list will occupy it. So, he has to keep it. He'll pay all his bills and I will pay mine. But we're still together, and he is my best friend."

Alex and Ana were having dinner that night, only the two of them. Phillip was visiting a friend in the building.

"Our lives have changed a lot," Ana said. "You know, we came to America for our daughter to have a safe, better life, to be sure she could live on her own. And now, when we see this happening, we aren't happy.

Maybe you are, but I am not. My English is not as good as it should be for college. Sarah will be living on her own. Life goes on, I know it, but it is so hard to accept all the changes."

"Of course, I agree with you. I worry and I'm terrified to know that our daughter in a wheelchair lives in such a huge city; it feels like a jungle sometimes. There are so many predators, and she has no idea how to protect herself. I wish she would live with Edmond. I feel like she would be much safer with a man than being alone. And your English will get better day by day; just be patient. Old people learn slower than the young ones."

"You call me old? Sometimes, you're right, I feel old! About Sarah, we have to get used to seeing her live by herself and be proud of her achievements. Why are we so sad? We have to change our mentality and let her spread her wings. How many handicapped people back in our country can do what Sarah does? She is a fighter; she will be ok. Of course, she is my girl."

* * * *

New York City never scared Ana, and she never felt the "culture shock." She came from a big city and that helped a little. Ana could spend days looking at the most beautiful decorated windows in the world, going to all the museums, or to the classical concerts. She enjoyed the big city life and Alex was enjoying it too, but in a different way. For him, the time spent outside, playing sports with his son was his idea of entertainment, enjoying every second of it. Connecticut and Long Island were his favorite places to go.

Ana remembered one day that would remain carved in her memory forever.

It was a weekend when all of them would be together and the Monday after, no one had to go to school or work. Alex was driving the big van they purchased for Sarah, to take her places. None of them knew where they were going, just to go somewhere, to be together. Suddenly, Ana saw a sign on the right side of the highway that said '360 miles to Montreal.' "Let's go to Montreal!"

"Ana, did you say Montreal?"

"Yes," she said. "Can we go?"

"Of course, but we have only our green cards and some money, no luggage."

"Who needs luggage?"

"Ok, you are right; let's go."

They went to Montreal and had the time of their lives. They bought necessary items for hygiene, nightgowns, and pajamas. What a memory! How precious it would be to remember years and years from now that they visited Toronto, Niagara Falls, had a good time, and returned home happy.

* * * *

"Alex, this morning I talked to St. Anthony at St. Patrick Cathedral. Actually, I've been going there every day of the week. I grab my coffee, drink it and the next stop, I go and pray and talk to him. I prefer him more than the other saints. Because, when I was pregnant with Phillip, I asked him for a baby boy and I had a baby boy. Later on, I asked about America, and I said that I would do everything he told me to do, and here we are, living in America. Many people would laugh if I told them what I just told you, but it is so true—I love him. So, today I asked him what to do with Phillip, what would be the best place to raise him well and safe. I know Sarah will be living in New York without us, and this is the only problem I see. I love this city, I adore this city, and it is so full of life. Ok, I talked too much."

"No, keep going. What is the end of your 'speech?' Do you want to move from here? Are you crazy? This would be my dream come true. You are always full of surprises. Nobody can get bored with you. Let me see what's new this time."

"All the money we make, and we make good money, goes to rent, parking, food, car repairs, and so many other bills; and we live in an apartment, not a house. What about moving somewhere where we can have a house and some trees around, a yard, something green. And feel more secure about raising our son in a better environment. I know you know how much I love this city, but it is time to consider other options for all of us."

"What about Sarah? She has to have the big city convenience, what she has here, and I don't think there are too many cities in this country offering such amazing things for people with a disability. It will be hard to find something similar, but we can try."

They used one of their vacations to explore the South. The main things that made them decide to look for a better place were Phillip's safety and Alex's chance to become a physical therapist. If Hunter College would accept his credits, he could enroll and graduate in a short period of time, considering he already graduated one college.

Moving to another state could be a huge, frightening thing. To start everything from scratch, no jobs, no friends, but they had to do it, to see Phillip attending a better school and to see Alex with a degree.

When Sarah heard the news, she knew this would be hard for her, but she trusted her parents to do the best they could for her. She even thought maybe Edmond would like it too; everything depended on the accessibility for disabled people. Sarah couldn't function without all the help she had now.

"Alex, if we like what we see over there, we may have to rent a house for quite some time to be sure this is what we are looking for. Otherwise, we can continue and live where we are now."

"I agree, but how can we do this? What about your job? I hope this college offers evening classes so I can work."

"There are spas and salons there too. I will find something to do. And if you can work and go to school, that would be great.

"You are just crazy again. How can we move somewhere without having something like a job, a house? Actually, we did it before, moving to a whole new country, and we did well. It seems that you love the unknown. Maybe we are gypsies!"

"No, I am too responsible to play like this, but I know what I know. My company has lots of beauty counters in Atlanta and they would be happy to offer me a job, bringing in the New York style. I am kidding, but I am a celebrity for my company."

"What about our daughter?"

"She will come and stay with us two, three times a year, and we'll fly there at least two times. That is only if we can't find something similar with what she has now. She told me she would do it, if we find it. She said that nobody has parents like she does and that she has to learn to live without my wings spread over her all the time."

* * * *

Alex spent days looking for the best schools for Phillip. He wanted his son to attend the best school, to get a good education.

They went to Atlanta, directly to the suburbs. They had no time to waste. The city seemed to be spread horizontally, and even if it was huge, it didn't look like it. There was so much green!

Everywhere they looked, it was full of trees, shrubs, bushes, plants. But at the same time, they noticed that everybody was driving; there were no sidewalks! It took them almost ten days to look for neighborhoods with good schools. The family found a house located within the best school's zip code. The house wasn't for sale, but they could rent it.

Phillip began easily at the school and immediately liked his classmates, making friends. But he kept saying that the family was not united without his sister. Sarah came to visit and explore the neighborhood; to see if she could live there. Ana knew the answer and felt guilty that she made such a change in their lives, to move without her daughter, who now lived hundreds of miles away.

She tried to convince herself that the move was a good thing for Sarah's future, giving her the opportunity to live independently, on her own—the main reason for coming to America. Ana kept her thoughts to herself, even though Alex had the same questions bothering him. Phillip was the only one saying loud and clear, what he thought about Sarah.

She spent a few days with the people she loved the most, and when the time came to go back to New York, she said, "Mom, you know better than me that I cannot live here. It's beautiful; I love the place you choose, but I didn't see sidewalks and everybody drives. I can't drive. I do have some good news, though. I'm seeing a different young man, named Jimmy. We became friends at school. H's disabled like I am, but he can stand and even walk with a walker. I cannot wait for you to meet him. He would like to become a broker. His family is like you, they love their children. He has a sister, and I like his family. Mom, I promise I will come to visit and you could come up there and stay with me. I miss Phillip more than I can say in words. I feel like I'm his mother."

"Sarah, I feel guilty by leaving you, but it was the only way to cut the umbilical cord! It was me that was keeping you like a prisoner. I had no strength to let you go."

"Mom, please don't ever talk like this! You sacrificed everything you had for me. How can you even think that? I love you so much."

They hugged each other and cried until they felt lighter and their hearts were healed.

The whole family took Sarah to the airport and everyone had a tough time saying goodbye. Ana looked at her daughter, how she pushed her manual wheelchair all the way to the security gate, and she felt like something died in her soul. She wanted to run, cross all the security lines, and help her. Tears were rolling down her cheeks and regret enveloped her. "Why, why?" she kept asking herself.

Sarah called them as soon as she arrived in New York and made Ana feel better.

Her daughter had her own life and she seemed to be happy.

CHAPTER FIFTEEN

It was time to look for a job, to make money. Ana called a few plastic surgeons' offices and got an appointment with a reputable one.

Unfortunately, Hurricane Opal hit the city and it took Ana two and a half hours to get to that interview. She knew she would get the job, but when she came home, she said, "I didn't move from the most beautiful city in the world to spend my entire life in traffic. I have to find something closer to the house, and I will."

The company she worked for in New York offered her a very high-paying salary to work at Neiman Marcus, where they had a beauty counter. Ana went and helped the company for a few days, being offered whatever she wanted, just to stay with them. The problem was the traffic. Ana wasn't going to accept it, even if she needed a stable job.

"Alex, let's go after dinner and look around our area, who knows what we can find. I am glad there are so many Jewish temples around us."

"What's the connection? I don't see it."

"Alex, Jewish husbands are taking care of their wives and their daughters. Do you remember how many Jewish ladies I had in New York? What good clients they were."

"Now, I see! Let's go, I'm ready when you are."

Phillip jumped in the car. He loved being with his father in the car, watching how he drove and learning the tricks his father knew.

Ana noticed a very elegant hair salon, not too far from their home. She grabbed a pen and wrote down the phone number listed on the window.

The next morning, she called the number, talked to the owner, and explained what she was looking for. The owner of the salon started laughing, saying that he tried to have some skin-care services for his clients, but it didn't work out. He invited Ana to come anyway. Ana went there, introduced herself, and the owner was happy to talk to her. He showed her the room that she could rent if she wanted.

Oh, my God, she thought, the room is the size of a small closet!

Ana agreed to rent it, and she was clear and firm from the beginning that she was going to open her own business soon and that she would be renting the space for a short period of time.

He seemed more than happy to get some money from a space that he didn't utilize, being sure she wouldn't make it, like all the other ladies that tried before her.

Ana was thankful to her mom every day for instilling the love for beauty in her heart. She couldn't wait for the next day to come so she could work.

* * * *

A year and a half went by, Alex and Ana bought a house that had what they wanted, near the best schools and in a family-oriented neighborhood. It seemed like their dream came true. They moved into the new house and shortly after that, house became home. It had so much love and care inside and everybody did what they could to make it feel amazing.

Ana went on a shopping spree, getting things to decorate. Most of the décor had a similar look to what they had back in Bucharest. Their home was peaceful, always a pleasure to come back from work and take a deep breath and relax. Even when there were many things to do around the house, it was still relaxing, because they loved it and they were happy to see the all the improvements done in the house. But they were missing their baby girl, even if they knew she was doing great and that their mission had been accomplished, to see her living independently.

Sarah was doing great and she was in love. "Mom, I love living here. This country is my paradise and it makes everything I do much easier. I can go to Manhattan any time I want; I can cross the bridge with my motorized wheelchair. I have to be sure I charge the battery the night before. It`'s amazing how many things a person in a wheelchair can do! Actually, I don't see too many differences between regular people and the disabled ones. This is my city, and I love it."

After listening to what her daughter had to say, Ana felt a huge sense of relief.

She knew things were getting better for everybody.

* * * *

Ana's work was giving her an immense feeling of satisfaction. The clients started to book her days in advance, and her boss was always trying to convince her to stay with him. Ana had other ideas. One day, she decided to share them with her husband.

"Alex, let's start making our own product line. I know how to do it, but we will need to invest some money."

"Ana, you're getting crazier and crazier every day! How in the world can you believe you can compete with the doctors? They have the skin-care products and the treatments exclusively. At least, I think so."

"You are wrong! Doctors can do whatever they want. The aesthetics services, what we, the aestheticians do is different. The approach is different and our services are a hundred years old. The doctors' are only a few years old. Believe me, we are going to do well. We will be successful and people will love our products; look how much they like what I do for them already."

Since he came to America, Alex has listened to his wife. He already found a job that required lots of lifting, but he was glad to bring money home. The college he wanted to attend was way too expensive; they couldn't pay such an enormous amount of money. Alex's dream of going to college had to be over.

Ana looked around her neighborhood to find a small place for lease, so she could open her business. There was a shopping center that looked rundown; the anchor store was out of business and there were only a few businesses open. She contacted the management company listed, and after a few discussions, Ana signed the lease. The first thing she did after signing the documents, was go to the shopping center and introduce herself to her neighbors.

One of them, a nice but tough German lady, looked at her and, instead of saying, 'nice to meet you,' she said, "Are you crazy? Nobody will survive here. Did you see what place you rented?"

Ana smiled and said, "Wait and see how this place will look and how many people will come to this plaza!"

· The German lady was the owner of a hair salon and had her business there for many years. She clearly thought Ana was out of her mind and that she would fail as soon as she opened her shop, but she wished her good luck.

Alex started working on the new place every day after coming home from work. He knew how to make all the repairs, and Phillip was like a full-time employee, working his tail off to help his father. What a blessed bond they had! Father and son were one team, working together, and you couldn't hope for a better, closer relationship. Phillip got his life teachings there. He put so many things in his mind and soul, connected with his father. Besides the fact, that he learned skills not too many teenagers had at his age.

Ana's heart was full of gratitude, thanking God for everything he was pouring over her family and her.

* * * *

When all the renovations were nearly done, when everything was ready to the smallest detail, a cabinet behind the reception desk fell and broke into pieces.

"Oh my God, I can't believe this. What are we going to do now?" Ana was desperate and started to cry.

"Do not worry. I will buy a cabinet tomorrow and install it."

"Yes, but we are going to open the doors officially tomorrow, and there will be a huge, ugly spot behind the reception desk."

"I have an idea. What about if you paint that space where the cabinet was in a contrast color, so it will look like it is a 'design'?"

"It sounds good to me. Let me get some paint and I will do it."

The next day, when the place opened for business, everything looked beautiful and it was a success. Ana received so many compliments for the spa and, especially, about that newly painted spot!

"Alex, I hope this business will make people happy and bring us money, so we can start working together. Your job is hard on your back, and we aren't getting younger."

"Oh no, I have to keep my job! Your trips to New York to see Sarah cost lots of money."

"I know you're right, but time will tell."

And time did tell. Their spa became the talk of their neighborhood; the clients were happy and they were coming back, bringing other friends, relatives, and neighbors. People were talking about their services, their products, their honesty, and their sincere approach.

"Alex, looking back, I think you were so right to call me crazy! I asked you to move to a part of the country where we didn't know a soul, beside my sister, and she recently moved here. Then on top of everything, to open a business with no money while took us six months to get the smallest loan the banks offered. I'm not blaming the bank; we are new to this country and we didn't have time enough to build up credit. I'm grateful we got the loan."

Just after Ana opened the spa, she got a call from Sarah.

"Mom, I wish I could be there with you for such an amazing event in our lives, but I have college papers to prepare. I wish you the best."

"Thank you, Sarah. I know. Otherwise, I would have bought you the air ticket, and you know that. You were present in my heart, like always. Your brother talks about you all the time and hopefully, you'll see each other soon."

"Mom, I miss all of you, but Phillip is the one I miss the most. I adore him."

"You always say this. I'm happy my kids love each other so

much."

"I will come down there as soon as I finish my last exam. Love you."

"Ok, try to give me the exact day, so I can purchase the ticket as soon as possible. The longer we wait the more expensive the ticket will be."

"I will call soon with that. Love you, Mom. Kiss Papa and Phillip for me."

That afternoon, Phillip came home happier than ever. "Mom, graduation is getting closer and I will need a tuxedo, new shoes, and a special white shirt. My date is gorgeous!"

"What does 'your date' mean? Is she your girlfriend?"

"Mom, I can see you have no idea what a date means, a date for the graduation doesn't have to be your girlfriend. She's gorgeous, and I know she will be very elegantly dressed."

"Son, you cannot complain that you don't have the most beautiful girls around you! It seems like all of them go to your school. 'm happy for you, and don't worry, you will be dressed very nicely. Son, did you feed the dogs?"

"Yes, ma'am, I did. Mom, do you remember when we moved from New York and after few days, I asked you to let me adopt a dog?"

"How is it possible to forget such a thing? I let you go to the Humane Society and your father let you adopt two dogs!"

"You know, Mom, they were sisters!"

"You keep saying the same thing for years. No, they were not sisters."

"Yes, they were in the same cage. I had to take them both. They were so beautiful, playful pups. I love them. This is one thing I love about living here. We couldn't have a dog in that New York apartment, but I miss my sister."

"You'll see her soon. I don't like leave too much time in between visits."

"I know and I cannot wait to see her. I love my sister."

* * * *

Graduation day came and Phillip was the most handsome guy from the entire group. Tall and slim with black eyes and black hair. And his light skin made a strong contrast.

Ana and Alex were grateful for another fact now becoming a reality. Their son would go to college and start a new life, a different life.

Ana watched her son during the ceremony, and remembered what happened when Philip told her that he was going to Panama City for his spring break. Ana had never heard these kind of words before—your child going on vacation by himself. What exactly was the meaning of what he said? She couldn't believe what she'd heard! She told a few clients about her son's intention to go to Panama City, for spring break. Everybody she talked to about Panama City, Florida, had the same reaction: "No, don't let him go. You have no idea what the teenagers do there. They drink alcohol till they drop dead, and some get arrested. Don't let him go there."

Ana went home and talked to her husband, sharing with him the things she found out about the city her son was going to. "Alex, our son is a young man now and we cannot stop him from going with his friends, but if something happens, I want to be there, close to him, just in case—to be sure he is ok."

"What do you mean? How can you be sure. How can you help if you are here and he will be there?"

"Oh no, that will not happen. We're going there too, but he doesn't have to know about our plan. He would be so embarrassed if his friends found out."

"No, we cannot do such a thing."

"Yes, we can. The spa will be very slow because everybody goes to the ocean for a week, so we'll go too. Let me make a reservation, as soon as I find out what hotel he's going to, and I will book one not too far from his."

Ana didn't say one word to Phillip, then for a full week, she and her husband were watching each step their son made while in Florida. They were on the beach, under an umbrella, and their eyes were on the pool where Phillip was hanging out with boys and girls. At the end of the week, Ana suggested driving around and looking at the real estate. Alex tried to convince her that they didn't have enough money to buy a house there, but Ana made an appointment with a real estate agent to show them a few houses.

On the last day of their "vacation," the agent told them there was one more house to show them and it was located on their way back home, close to the bridge. Both of them agreed to see the last house on the list. The moment they arrived, Ana's heart was beating faster—she just loved it.

Alex knew it right away, when he saw his wife's reaction.

Ana and Alex went back to their home and started making calculations, to see how they could pay for a second mortgage!

They purchased that house in the same year of Phillip's graduation. If Phillip hadn't gone for spring break, they wouldn't have that beautiful house. They'd never been to Florida before; the only thing they knew was work, and only work.

It seemed like things were getting so much better, with their daughter living on her own and being independent. Their son was going to start college soon and the business was doing really well—so well, in fact, that they had three salons now!

Ana couldn't believe how much strength she had, being able to run three spas and being responsible for so many aestheticians, training, products, clients, and all the things that come along with being a business owner.

Alex was going from one place to another, fixing equipment, making products, dealing with all the paperwork, the accountant, everything.

They couldn't be more grateful, but everyone knows that even the best things must come to an end.

"Ana, can you come here please?" Alex said.

"Ok, what is it?"

"Look at these red spots. What do you think?"

"Do they itch? Hurt?"

"No," Alex answered.

Ana didn't like what she heard. If those red spots don't itch and don't hurt, that wasn't a good sign. "Let me call my dermatologist, the one that I work with."

Ana worked very closely with a reputable dermatologist and she loved Ana. She asked Ana to work for her in her medical practice and Ana helped her for a few months before she opened her own spa. Ana recommended this doctor for any skin problems, trusting her with all her clients. She called and made an appointment. When the doctor found out who called, she grabbed the phone and told Ana to come right away, don't wait.

Alex showed the doctor what the problem was and the doctor recommended Emory Hospital, saying that she didn't have the necessary equipment Alex would need.

Ana knew right away that something wasn't right. She knew it was a bigger problem. "Thank you, Doctor, I will call and make the appointment today."

"No, you need to go there today. I want your husband to start the treatment today, if that's possible."

"It is that bad?"

"Yes, but he has a chance. This isn't a joke, Ana. Let me know if I can help and I will, you know this. Your husband needs special ultraviolet rays and a few more other treatments that I don't have here in the clinic. This hospital is better equipped and I trust their treatments. They have excellent doctors as well. It's a teaching hospital."

"My husband has never been sick, not even the flu!" Ana tried to convince her that it had to be a mistake, that her husband couldn't be sick…he was too strong.

The conversation was taking place outside the office, when Alex was getting dressed. As soon as they got back to work, Ana called the doctor and she was so happy to make an appointment for the next day.

They went to the hospital and Alex had many blood tests done.

"Ana, the doctor called me," Alex said after checking out one of their clients.

"What did she say?"

"She wanted me to start the treatment 'last week,' before I saw her! I thought she was joking, and she said I have leukemia, stage four."

"What? Is she crazy? You cannot have cancer; you're too healthy, too strong. Do you remember when she decided to have one more test done, after everything came back perfect? She was sure that it was just a superficial epidermal condition, but then she changed her mind, asking for that extra test. God spoke through her voice. I still hope it is a mistake, somebody else's blood." She tried to fool her brain, but the result came back positive.

"Ana, I have cancer and she wants me to start chemotherapy right away. She said that the last blood test she'd ordered brought the results she was talking about. I'm not scared. I am only concerned about you and the kids. How can you handle all the things we have to do?"

"This should be the last thing on your mind. I will be with you day and night, and I will make arrangements at work, so somebody will take care of things."

Alex was scheduled to have the "port" implanted on his upper chest. When this procedure was done, he had an appointment with the doctor that was going to be "his" doctor.

A young doctor came into the room; you could easily see that he never went to a gym. So young, that Ana didn't like to the idea of him being her husband's doctor, but something calmed her down and she listened to what he had to say. The doctor examined Alex, checked his folder and all the blood results, then he pulled a chair closer to Alex and said, "Considering how fit and young you are and the fact that you have never been sick, I think you have a ten percent chance to get this in remission. The disease you have been diagnosed with is a deadly disease; it is at stage four. I do have to inform you from the beginning that the treatment that I will prescribe for you is the most powerful chemotherapy somebody can get. There's no other treatment that I know about, and we have to start now."

Alex liked his doctor; he was scared, but nobody could see this on his face.

"Alex, you stay here and start the treatment like the doctor says. I will go home, take care of the dogs and I'm not sure if Phillip will be home from school. Then, I will go to work and take care of things. Don't worry; everything will be ok. I will be back after six tonight and stay with you for the night. I'll bring you some food from home because I know how you are."

"Oh no, stay home. I will be ok."

"No, I will be with you like I said." Ana went to her spa and made arrangements for the next couple of weeks to transfer her clients to other aestheticians, so they wouldn't miss their beauty treatments.

After finishing what she had to do at the spa, she went home to check on her son and the dogs. Phillip jumped up and hugged his mother with so much love that Ana almost started to cry. How good it was to feel loved.

"Mom, how is Dad doing? What did the doctor say?"

"The doctor gave hope to your father, but he has to get through those horrible chemo sessions. Your dad cannot eat because of the chemo, but I'll prepare something very light for him. Now I'm sorry I didn't teach you how to cook. You will need it now. I regret I can't spend more time with you, son. This was my regret since we came to America. I should be home when you come from school. Did you talk to your sister today?"

"Not yet. You told me not say one word about Dad's situation, to keep my mouth shut."

"I know what I told you, but you can talk to her about anything else. We have to know how she is doing, because there's always something with her. There is not a day that goes by without me wondering how she can live there, by herself and without asking for financial help. Of course, we send her packages and sometimes money, but she never asked for it. Son, do you think that coming to America was a good thing?"

"No question!" Phillip answered promptly. "Look how many things Sarah can do by herself! She can go everywhere she wants, anytime she wants."

"What about you? Are you happy?"

"I feel like I was born here. No one even guesses that I'm Romanian."

"You are, but now you are an American citizen. Your language is better than all of us put together. You have no accent."

"Mom, I am amazed by Sarah, but at the same time. I am mad with her."

"What? I never heard you being mad at your sister. It must be serious. What do you know that I don't know?"

"She has to do something to improve her physical condition. The powered wheelchair is excellent, but now she relies on it too much! I understand it is easier, but she has to build up some muscles, to be able to transfer from the wheelchair to her bed, and so many other things she should do. But now, you are in a hurry; we'll talk later."

"I am cooking, so we can talk."

"You know, it is hard and it is a lot of work for her, but if she doesn't do it now, later on it will be harder. Look at me, if I miss two days going to the gym, my body feels it."

"I know, but do you remember what I told you about working out so much? I know you do, because I keep saying it all the time. It is very important to work out your body, but it is more important, or, at least, equally important, to train your brain. Am I right? You must be tired of how many times I told you this."

"Mom, I like having strong muscles. Are trying to say that I'm not smart?"

"Son, this has to be impossible. You are my son; you have to be smart."

Phillip was glad that his mom was able to joke and smile, considering what she had to go through. Both of them had a tiny break from the avalanche of sadness, diseases that were coming their way. "Mom, I'll get to the hospital after the rush hour. I will see you later on. How much longer do you think dad will be in the hospital?"

"Do you remember what the doctor said? Your father's disease is a deadly one. A stage four cancer is deadly, but considering his physical condition and the fact that he was never sick, the doctor gave him a ten percent chance of surviving. It's bad, very bad. But do you know something? Our prayers, our faith, and our love will save your father's life. It has to. We all need him in our lives, but one thing… Sarah doesn't have to find out. She has an inclination for depression, and that's all she needs. We have to come up with a plan, an idea, for how to tell her and when. Sarah would give her life for her father."

"Me, too!"

Ana knew the meaning of her son's words. The truth had been spoken and it made Ana's heart full of love for her family.

Ana remembered the time when she and her brother were taking care of their younger sister, Sophia. They loved taking care of her, playing together, teaching her things, and all the love they had for her. Just thinking of her sister and her brother, tears were coming into her eyes.

Love is painful, even when you're happy. But what about now, when the entire world is down for her and her family? *How can we fight a monster like cancer? How is it possible for the world to be so advanced, to fly to the moon, and not have a cure for cancer?*

Ana was trying to see a reason; why did they have to suffer? Cancer didn't affect just one person; cancer affected all those that love the person with cancer, too. *I'm feeling sick now, and I have no physical pain. Just my soul that's hurt and weeping. I have to fool my brain.* Ana remembered a very smart passage written by a philosopher saying that you have to repeat a few words a few times a day that can change your life: "Day by day, from all points of view, I feel better and better." And she promised to do it.

"I will get stronger. I will be a fighter; my family needs me more than ever," Ana was repeating her "motto" to educate her brain and get strength for the fight she had to be ready for. Back then, her God didn't hold as much meaning for her as he should. Ana had no religious education. She couldn't believe her love for God was so real when she never learned about it in school, but her family gave her the love for God, and she was adding daily proof. Even if she didn't need any proof to believe in him. Ana knew the book of her life was already written and the book was in God's library. Every day was like turning a page, without knowing what the next page would bring.

Now, Alex's disease seemed to start a new chapter of their lives, an unwanted chapter, a painful one, full of struggles and hopes.

All those thoughts were chasing Ana's mind. She took care of the employees, the clients, and things seemed to be ok. Ana was blessed with amazing coworkers, and everybody was ready to help.

* * * *

The first week of chemo was over, and the doctor told Ana that she could take Alex home to recover after the horrible chemo sessions. Her husband was very weak and extremely pale. Alex was so happy to go home, to sleep in his own bed. He even asked Ana to give him the car keys. "Ana, I want to drive!"

"Are you sure you can? You went through so much; you have no strength."

"I know, but it makes me happy to drive again."

Ana gave him the car keys and started praying to God to get home safely. Everything it was ok until they hit the highway! The traffic was bumper-to-bumper, and the smell of the pollution, the intoxicated air, the poison of the pollution, made Alex so sick that they had to pull over and figure out the back roads to get home.

Alex looked at his home, played with the dogs—so happy to see them. "Ana, it feels so good to be home. I wish I didn't have to go back."

"Ok, let's not think about it for a week. You need good food and rest. This is what the doctor told me, so I will be your nurse."

The moment Phillip came home, he didn't let his father alone; he was at his father's side all the time. Ana had to invent new food, to try and see if Alex could take it. That chemo changed the way he tasted food, the way he smelled things, and it was only the first round of chemo; four more to go.

Alex couldn't eat but at least he tasted some. "Ana, I can't eat, but maybe tomorrow I will be better."

Poor Phillip had to eat all his mother's inventions, all the new food.

* * * *

"Ana, wake up; wake up, fast! I'm having a heart attack! I have excruciating pain in my arms. Please, wake up."

Ana was so exhausted from all the work during the day that her sleep was so deep she didn't hear all the things Alex was telling her, but she realized something bad must have happened. She went downstairs and called the ambulance, turned the lights on like she'd been instructed to do by the operator, grabbed some warm clothes, and stayed next to Alex. There was nothing she could do; his pain was making his entire body struggle with spasms.

The pain was something he'd never experienced before in his life. The ambulance took them to the nearest hospital. At least, this is what they said to Ana. It was forty minutes away from their house, and even if it was three o'clock in the morning, there was still traffic.

The moment they arrived at the hospital, the nurses did an unbelievable job. Ana never saw that kind of professionalism; everybody knew exactly what to do. One of the nurses came and asked questions necessary for the doctor. When she heard about chemo and especially what kind of chemo Alex had, she looked at Ana like she was seeing a widow. But very calmly, she invited Ana to go to the waiting room and sit down, promising that somebody would come and talk to her as soon as they could.

"Ma'am, we did the best we could. Now we're waiting for the doctor. He will come shortly."

"To come from where? There's no doctor in the emergency room? How is this possible?"

"He is on call, and he will be here in a moment." The nurse apologized for not having a doctor there, in the emergency room, knowing that it could cost the patient's life.

Ana thought she was living in a nightmare. This couldn't be real; it was something she'd never heard about. She went to the waiting room and started talking to God, in her way. Her prayers were just telling God what was in her mind. It was a very cold November night. She tried to close her eyes, but the long hallway was so frightening, she was scared to be alone. She would prefer to be with Alex.

Suddenly, she heard footsteps on the floor and noticed a man walking slowly towards the emergency room. Ana couldn't help but think, *whoever is waiting for this doctor, I assume he is a doctor, had plenty of time to die!* The man had a suitcase that looked like the ones doctors had.

Little did she know, that man was Alex's surgeon. It took him forty-five minutes to get to the hospital, who knows from where. Ana made the connection when "that man" came to talk to her, this time, wearing a white jacket.

He introduced himself and said, "I just finished putting a stent in your husband's artery. Everything went well and I am going to see him later. I was informed about the cancer treatment and the type of chemo he is under. Mr. Alex has to wait for his heart to get stronger, because now only twenty-five percent of his heart is working. In order to be able to receive the next round of chemo, he has to get stronger."

"Thank you, sir. We will do what has to be done."

"My nurse is going to inform his cancer doctor, and I have to see your husband for a follow-up in a week."

The next day, Ana and Alex went home.

Phillip was so happy to see his father back home.

"How could you do this to me?" Ana asked her husband, even though she was grateful he was alive. It was just a way to talk to him, to make him stronger. In other words, he wasn't allowed to be sick; he had to live. He had to be there with his family.

"Ana, if I get a heart attack after each chemo session, I won't last long. The chemotherapy was so poisoning that it tore my artery, so now I have a stent in my heart. I won't go back to the hospital."

"You see, this is your biggest problem. Everything you see is black; I see pink. You have to change the way you think. These things are connected—you know better than me; you went to college."

"Are you making fun of me?"

"No, but I can see you dying. You have no right to leave me with a daughter in a wheelchair and a son that needs his father, two dogs, a business, a house, and me! No, you are not allowed to die. I will make you change the way you think and you'd better know how stubborn I am."

"I promise you, this cancer it will be gone; it has to be gone. I've had enough of tragedy in my life, and do you know something? God is on our side; we will make it."

* * * *

They went for the follow-up appointment with the heart doctor, and he said, "I spoke with your cancer doctor, and we put together a treatment plan for you. Next week, you can start your second round of chemo. You will be fine."

"Thank you, Doctor, but how do I know I won't have another heart attack after the next chemo?"

"Nobody knows it, but your heart is functioning well right now and the stent I put in, it will help. Good luck and I'll see you for the next follow-up."

The second round of chemotherapy treatment started strong. The side effects were horrible. Alex could smell the food from a distance, making him sick to his stomach. The doctor said it would be the most toxic chemo they have.

One of the nurses brought Ana a pillow and a blanket so she could sleep a little on the only chair in the room. The equipment used all the space in Alex's room; and all the monitors, the nurses coming every thirty minutes or so—everything was depressing, but Ana had to keep her thoughts positive. She had to show her husband she was strong and that she was ready to do whatever it would take to see him well.

Five full days, twenty-four hours a day, the toxic chemo ravaged Alex's body.

She could see the changes in his appearance, in a bad way.

"I never thought I would be in this situation, even the smell of food makes me sick. This second round of chemo is a strong poison," Alex said to his wife. "I have no desire to wake up in the morning, if I sleep during the night. Most of the time, I cannot sleep. I am nauseated. The food makes me sick."

Ana let him talk, and she knew that she had a special role in his recovery; she had to be strong for both of them. Then she remembered. "Oh, how could I forget about Sarah? She'll be here next week. I bought an air ticket for her a long time ago and completely forgot about it. Can you believe it? How am I going to tell her about the situation, about you? I can't be the one to tell her. I cannot do this. Phillip will do a much better job than me. I will let him talk to her. Who is going to help her with the shower in our home? Phillip can't do this; he's a man. Who's going to stay with her in the house when I am with you in the hospital? It's not like before when I was taking her with me to the spa and spending the whole day together. I have to cancel the ticket and ask her to come in the spring."

"For what reason? She never missed a Christmas!"

Ana started crying. To see her crying was almost an event; she always put on such a strong face. "Ok, I can handle it, but I will let Phillip talk to her about your situation."

"I'm glad you changed your mind," Alex said. "Let her come. Who knows if I will see her again?"

In normal circumstances, Ana would be furious to hear what Alex said, but what if he was right?

CHAPTER SIXTEEN

"Phillip, your sister will be here in a few days and I need ask you to talk to her about your father's situation, please."

"Of course, I'll do it, but I'm so afraid of her reaction. She loves Dad so much. I have to think about this, to come up with a plan. Mom, I hate to do this."

"I know, but you're the only one that can talk to her."

Phillip went to the airport to wait for his sister. The plane arrived on time even if it was a snowy day. He saw her coming with a huge smile on her face. It was Sarah's gift; that is what she called her visits home. A gift to see her family, to spend time together. It was a sacred time, and a happy time.

As soon as they hugged each other, her first question was, "Where is Papa? He always waits for me; he's never missed being here to pick me up. Is he hiding? Is this a joke?"

"Let's have a coffee; I know how much you like coffee."

"Are you sure he isn't here, or is he waiting for us at the coffee shop?"

"No, he had some things to do."

"Do you know something, I don't believe you. My papa would leave anything he had going and he would come and wait for me at the airport. Is he ok? Is Mom ok? Oh, I know she is, I just talked to her. But I haven't talked to Papa for a long time and you know, for us, even a week is a long time."

They had coffee together, even though Phillip wasn't crazy about coffee, but he needed time to figure out when to start and how to start telling his sister about the deadly disease their father was fighting.

Phillip helped his sister transfer from her wheelchair to the car seat, folded the wheelchair, and put it in the trunk. Every movement he made was so slow; trying to postpone "the talk."

"I'm so glad you came, Sarah. I missed you. I have some friends, and all of them have siblings, so I feel lonely without you."

"Hey, are you ok? You never talk like this, you're always in a hurry, and I barely spend time with you! What's going on? Everything is so strange!"

"Sarah, our dad would never miss waiting for you at the airport; you're right about that. Our dad is in the hospital with cancer, but he will be ok, I promise." Phillip had no idea how the last sentence came out of his mouth. He had to say it then he thought his sister would faint. He couldn't stop her tears all the way to the hospital.

Once they arrived there, it was like a choir of tears. The moment Sarah saw her father lying down on the hospital bed, with tubes all over and his head bald, she started screaming, and her tears were making everybody cry.

"Papa, don't die! I love you."

"Don't worry, I will live forever." Alex smiled and hugged his daughter as much as his tubes and Sarah's wheelchair let them.

Ana let them be together. She knew her daughter's love was in front of her; she had eyes only for her papa. Ana grabbed her paperwork and went to a tiny corner of the room. She hated the paperwork, which was the kind of work usually done by Alex. She didn't want to touch it, but now she had to. The business had to pay the taxes, the accountant, and the salaries for their employees. She tried to concentrate on what she had to do, but it was impossible. She closed her eyes and let her mind talk to her.

* * * *

"Sarah, it's time to go home; your dad has to get some rest."

"He can rest. I will stay here with him."

"Where are you going to sleep?"

"In my wheelchair."

Ana and Phillip went home and let Sarah spend the night with her papa. The nurses told Ana that everything would be ok, and if Sarah needed help, they would help her. The bathroom was large and wheelchair accessible. Nobody could convince Sarah to leave her father.

The next day, Phillip brought Sarah home to take a shower and change her clothes.

Ana was waiting for her children to sit down and have dinner. It was hard to make her leave, but she had to shower. She tried not to think about the rest of the bad news she had. "Sarah, do you remember that I purchased your ticket round trip, like always? Originally, you were supposed to go back to New York in a month, but this time, you have to leave earlier. I'm so sorry to say it, but I have to focus on your father."

"Not only that, but you have to take care of so many other things, too. I understand, but I am devastated. Tell me he will survive; tell me he will live, please?"

"He will, I promise. Nobody can die if I am in charge." Ana smiled.

"Mom, don't feel sorry for me. I am ok, but I'm very sad."

Sarah went back to her apartment, but she was miserable. Phillip and Ana called her every day to be sure she was ok and to tell her how her papa was doing. Both Phillip and Ana lied a lot about Alex's condition to protect her from the pain.

Ana had moments when she felt guilty about letting Sarah live alone in the big city. Many times, she asked herself if she'd made the right decision when they moved away from her, that they should have stayed together and been a family. But now she knew for sure that was the best thing she did. Her daughter could take care of herself; she continued to live there and go ahead with her own life. The big city was an oasis for Sarah. She could go everywhere she wanted; she was *independent*—and this was the magic word in Ana's mind.

Alex had to go three more times to the hospital for three more chemo sessions, five full days each. He was unrecognizable; his head was bald, no eyebrows, and his skin looked ashy. Ana was doing more than anybody could do to keep him alive. Her soul was so hurt that she was afraid she would be the next patient. Sometimes it was too much, even for her.

Communism, the death of her father, her mother's new marriage, moving three, four times a year to follow her stepfather with his job. Then almost losing her daughter to a government institution, immigrating to a country where she had no idea how they would survive there, struggling to make it, and now her husband's disease—plus a lot more less painful events in between.

Ana tried to convince herself that all the other "less painful" events were less painful indeed; but she knew, deep inside, that they were as painful as all the others. She remembered when her husband couldn't accept the horrible future that was inevitable by having a handicapped child, and he tried to find a "normal, peaceful" place.

You don't choose your life; it is given to you, and you have to do the best you can with it. And so she did.

* * * *

Alex was getting better day by day.

He was currently scheduled to have his blood cleaned up and his stem cells frozen.

Ana didn't understand much, but she witnessed each step of the sophisticated treatment. The machine Alex was connected to collected his blood and separated the stem cells through a centrifuge. It was a four-hour treatment and he wasn't allowed to move, not even an inch.

When Ana looked at the technology, the machine, the equipment the hospital had, she felt proud of her tax money! It seemed that they served a noble cause. She couldn't believe how "lucky" they were to have this happen in America. Even if they loved their country, they knew it would be impossible to be cured; impossible for the doctors to save your life. And not because of the knowledge, but because of the funds the regime didn't want to spend on such life-saving equipment. This was another way God showed them they were on the right path.

Alex was finally ready to have his own stem cells transplanted into his body.

After finishing the transplant, the nurses took Alex's blood for testing every couple of hours. They expected to see more of the red cells coming from his stem cells. Ana could see the disappointment in their eyes; the number had to be a lot higher than it was.

Imagine their surprise, when one of the nurses came into the room shouting with happiness, "Sir, I have never seen such an increase in numbers like I see on your tests. The last one came back with fantastic figures. Your cells grew by thousands! I can't wait to let the doctor know."

Ana and Alex didn't understand much, and it sounded like a new, different language, but seeing the nurse's face and her happiness, made them realize something good had happened.

Indeed, the doctor came in and he congratulated Alex. "Mr. Alex, there is no evidence of any cancer cells in your body. I can say you have entered remission! I'm thrilled to make this statement: the ten percent chance I gave you in the beginning has been turned into a hundred percent. You are cured, congratulations."

Ana jumped up, hugged the doctor, and said, "Doctor, I know it was my cooking, not your treatment!"

They all had a good laugh and Ana could see tears in her husband's eyes.

Alex was given his life back. "Doctor, thank you from the bottom of my heart. You worked so hard to save my life. Thank you."

A new life began! The home, the dogs, everything around Alex seemed so different, so new, like he never saw these things before. Everything had a new meaning, a new purpose. There were things he never paid attention to before he got sick, and now they were new to him. He had a new appreciation for everything. Alex always believed in God, but now he could feel God in his blood. It didn't take long and he started doing things like the cancer never happened.

Sarah couldn't be happier. "Sarah, we called you to let you know that your father entered remission and there are no traces of cancer cells in his blood."

"Mom, I am the happiest woman on Earth. My father is a strong man; I knew it. I cannot wait to come and see him. Now it will be a normal visit, like before, and I expect him to wait for me at the airport. How is everybody doing? Finally, I can ask my regular questions."

They talked for a while, and when she heard her father's voice, she couldn't finish the conversation. The tears took her voice away. Alex tried a few times to talk to his daughter, but he had to give up.

Later on, Sarah called back and she was able to enjoy talking to her papa. She told him that her boyfriend, Jimmy, asked to marry her, but she wasn't sure she wanted to be married, at least not yet. His mother loved Sarah and she wished her son would marry Sarah. But Sarah felt it wasn't her decision to make.

"Sarah, when you will feel ready, you'll know it. We like him, but it is you who needs to decide. Let us know. We love you."

When Alex went back to work, he was amazed at how well the girls took care of the business. There were no complaints, the clients were happy, the products were on the shelves, and he knew his son had worked on it.

They used the house they bought in Florida once in a while; sometimes for a weekend, to recharge their batteries. Ana always wanted to rent the house, so they could make more money, but Alex and the kids were always against her idea.

She had a practical, business-oriented mind; the others were dreamers.

It was around this time when the economy was crashing, but the home prices were ridiculously high, very high. Ana made a fast calculation in her mind and she knew they could sell the house for three times the price they paid for it. She approached her family, explaining that they could buy another house in the same area and pocket some money for retirement.

Oh my God, what she started. Sarah cried, Phillip was really sad, and Alex looked petrified.

He came right out and asked, "How could you come up with such an idea? You said you love this house."

"I do, but I can love another house too. Let's sell it. We will never be offered such prices again. The house market is a volcano. I only have to open my mouth, and the house would be sold."

"Please, stop talking like this. Nobody agrees with your idea."

It was the first time Ana couldn't win against her family. She was so used to seeing them doing whatever she wanted, but this house meant a lot to each of them. The house was medium sized but located in a very quiet, peaceful neighborhood. They couldn't see the water, being a more than hundreds of feet from the coast, but the house had a charm. It was very welcoming. The moment you opened the door, the fragrance, the flowers, everything was saying: welcome. It made you feel relaxed before even sitting on the sofa.

Ana tried to explain to her family all the benefits they could have from selling the house and buying a different one, but their ears were deaf.

"Ok, if that's the situation, let's move to the ocean, to retire."

The day Alex was declared cured, he dreamed about moving there, and really enjoyed the fishing. He didn't say much, but he was dreaming day and night about living there. He was afraid that his wife would think he'd lost his mind as they had a big business to run, and they had responsibilities. Everybody that worked for them had families, children to take care of. Ana would think he had a new disease developing—this time in his brain, God forbid!

Alex's dream was to move to the ocean, and Ana knew it. It amazed her how God arranged things, even if you don't want them to happen. She'd thought about moving already, but she didn't want to be like a gypsy, moving all the time. She already had roots in Atlanta; she had things she was responsible for.

* * * *

One of Ana's coworkers, Anastasia, was one of the most beautiful ladies Ana ever worked with. She was tall and thin, with huge eyes and a big heart. She approached Ana at work and said, "I checked your appointments and you have a few minutes free between clients. Do you mind if I talk with you during this time?"

Ana already felt upset. The first thing that came to her mind was that her aesthetician wanted to resign, to go to another place. "Of course, I will see you then." Ana didn't remember how she worked on her next client, she felt so anxious about it.

Anastasia entered the room and said, "You know how much I appreciate working with you and all the things you taught me. Everything I know is from you."

"Thank you for saying this. I appreciate working with you very much. All our clients love you. We worked together for almost ten years now."

"Ana, I talked to my husband. We know all the things you went through with Alex, his health and how hard it was for you to handle everything. I have an offer, and if you don't want to answer it now, I would wait until you can. My husband and I would like to buy your business."

"What? The business isn't for sale, but I am so happy you would consider buying it. I will talk to Alex, and who knows? I cannot say anything now. I'm shocked. But I promise I will talk to my husband."

"I know you make the decisions…I do too, but we have to ask our husbands, to have peace of mind."

"Yes, this is an important decision. It would be a life-changing decision, and I want him to be the one to say yes or no."

"Smart like always. Let me know what he says, please," she said, leaving the office.

The other girls were curious, thinking that their coworker was in trouble.

* * * *

Ana could barely hold in the joy when she got home. "Alex, we could sell the business and move to the ocean, like you want."

"Something is really wrong with you today. These aren't the kind of jokes I want to hear. How did you come up with this? You always have something new to say; every time you come home, you have stories to tell."

"Ok, this isn't a story. It is serious and I have to give an answer as soon as possible. Anastasia wants to buy our business. I have no other details to share with you. It was unexpected and it took me by surprise, but I like it."

"So, it is real?"

"Yes, and we have to come up with a price, to calculate everything, to make a decision, black or white. The time I spent with you in the hospital, the girls realized they could take care of the business by themselves, and this would be a great thing for us. I am very grateful."

"I couldn't have better news than this. I'll sleep like a baby tonight. I see myself already fishing."

Sarah and Ana kept in touch with each other daily. Being in the wheelchair, Ana was worried about her daughter crossing the busy boulevards, the bridges and she wanted to be sure Sarah got home safely.

"How are you, my dear?" Ana asked her daughter.

"I'm ok, I think."

"What do you mean 'I think'? Are you sick?"

"No, but there's something on my left side, I think it is part of my stomach, that bothers me."

"What does 'bother me' mean? Sarah, please be more specific. Do you have pain? Sharp or dull? Is your stomach swollen or flat? Tell me."

"I have some pain, but not all the time. I feel like something is pressing on my bladder."

"Did you see a doctor?"

"No, but I will make an appointment, and I'll let you know what he said, I promise. I know how you are. If I don't call, you'll come here right away."

"Correct, so don't make me fly, it costs lots of money. You better call and tell me what the doctor said. Love you."

"Oh, you just said 'love you!' Do you think I'm going to die? When you say 'I love you' it must be something special."

"I agree. If you keep saying 'love you' every time you talk to somebody, it becomes like 'hi, how are you?' Love is a very special word, for me at least."

"You're right like always. I love you, Mom, and I promise again I will call you as soon as I find out something."

Ana hung up the phone and her mind started spinning. "God, not again! I feel like something isn't right. Let me be wrong."

* * * *

Sarah made the appointment with the doctor, as she promised to her mother. The doctor ordered an ultrasound to "see" better what was going on inside Sarah's stomach.

"Mom, the doctor was right. There is a mass the size of a golf ball growing on my uterus. His office already scheduled a biopsy. I'm so scared."

"Don't be! You know your mom will be there for you, with you."

"Thank you. You are always here for me."

Ana purchased a round trip ticket so she could be back in two days; there were so many things she had to take care of at home. She had a "people business" to run, and people need people. She had to be there for her clients and for her coworkers. Alex never liked to be alone without his wife. The food was always almost untouched when she got back home. But now, Sarah was again, the priority.

Ana waited in the waiting room of the surgery department and was so happy to see Sarah come out of the surgery room. "Did it hurt?" she asked.

"A little, but I'm afraid it will be cancer. Mom, I'm so scared."

"No. It is not cancer. I know it."

"How do you know?"

"I know it because I am a mother, and mothers know everything. It is just a small tumor. The doctor will remove it, and everything will go back to normal." Ana tried to make her daughter smile.

"It sounds good to me. I'm tired of so many surgeries."

"Ok. Let's go to your apartment and I will cook a few dishes for you, so there will be no more ordering food."

"Thank you so much. You know how much I enjoy your

cooking."

Ana cleaned and cooked and felt really good helping Sarah. The next morning, she headed to the airport to catch her flight. Alex was waiting for her, happy to see his wife and to take her back home. The airport was an hour and a half away from their home and Alex had plenty of time to ask all the questions he wanted to have answers to. Ana explained about the biopsy, about the tumor, the schedule of the surgery, and they talked a lot about Sarah and her problems.

"Ana, let's pray the tumor is benign and she will recover fast from the surgery. Actually, you said that it will be done laparoscopic, am I right?"

"Yes, it is a simple procedure, but to me it is still surgery."

"You always get things complicated in your mind. She will be ok. The dogs missed you a lot. They stayed close to the door, facing the door, the whole time since you left. They are such smart dogs, and they know when something is going on. It felt so good to have a soul in the house to talk to. I don't like when you're not home. Everything is lifeless, too quiet, when you aren't there to stir things up. How long do you think it will take to get the results from the biopsy?"

"A couple of days, not too long, but for me it is too long."

They got home and the dogs were the happiest ever, jumping and running around Ana. What a good feeling, what a joy to come home and to see all the love waiting for you. Ana's home wasn't big or impressive, but it had something that most homes don't have: a soul! Her home was a temple of faith, hope, and love. She talked to and kissed her flowers and all the artwork she had; it had a meaning, a history and it served a purpose.

"Alex, it feels so good to be home. Let's have dinner, and after that, I'll call Sarah to see how she is doing."

They had a quick dinner, being late, and Ana called Sarah. "Hi, Sarah, how are you? Did you eat?"

"Not much. I'm not feeling well."

"What do you mean? What's wrong?"

"I think I have some fever."

"Did you take your antibiotics?"

"What antibiotics? I never got a prescription when I left the hospital!"

"Are you sure?"

"Yes, I am. The nurse didn't say anything about taking antibiotics."

"Can you please, check with your pharmacy, maybe they called in the prescription? You have to have antibiotics after the biopsy. I remember them saying so. They forgot to mention it to you, but I am positive they sent it to the pharmacy."

"You might be right. Let me call them, and I will call you back."

"Ok. I'll wait for your call." Ana was getting more worried by the minute; she was scared that her daughter got an infection from the biopsy.

Sarah called her mom back and said there was no prescription with her name at the pharmacy.

"You should call the nurse that released you and tell her about the fever."

"I will and call you back."

Ana was waiting, but she knew that it would take time for the nurse to call Sarah back, and Ana already sensed that Sarah wasn't doing well.

"Hi, Sarah, how are you? Did you talk to the nurse?"

"No, I left a message on her voicemail, but nobody called me yet."

"What about the fever?"

"It's going up, and I have chills. I am not well. Sorry, Mom, I don't want to bother you. You have so many things on your plate."

"Sarah, you should go back to the hospital and tell them the situation. It isn't safe to be home with fever, after the biopsy. Thank God, the hospital is so close to your apartment. I will call you there; they will connect us. And I will talk to you later on."

Sarah went back to the hospital, to the emergency room, where she was admitted right away. The fever had skyrocketed and they associated the high fever with an infection at the biopsy site.

Ana called the hospital and was told about Sarah's condition. The nurse explained to Ana that Sarah developed an infection and they were trying to get the fever down. Ana wanted to scream at her, blaming her for the lack of care—no antibiotics, nothing, letting her go home without medication! But she was calm, and she begged the nurse to take care of her baby girl.

"Alex, I am going back to New York now, tonight. Sarah has a high fever and she has an infection at the place they did the biopsy. I should get a flight attendant's job, that's how often I fly."

"Like always, there isn't much I can say. Let me take you to the airport."

* * * *

Ana arrived in New York and the taxi took her directly to the hospital where Sarah was. Not even in her worst nightmares could Ana imagine seeing her daughter looking like she did. Sarah was hallucinating, not recognizing her mother or knowing where she was! In a relatively short period of time, the high fever devastated Sarah's body. She was unrecognizable. She was shaking with chills and looking like a ghost.

Ana threw her purse on the floor and asked for towels and sheets. The personnel thought she was losing her mind, seeing her daughter so ill, but they gave her what she asked. Ana soaked the sheets and the towels in cold water and wrapped them around Sarah's body. After few more minutes, she repeated the wrapping. Ana asked to talk to a doctor about her daughter's condition and what has to be done. She was desperate.

"Please, explain to me, what's going on with my daughter. Why the fever doesn't go down? Why wasn't she given antibiotics after the biopsy?"

"Sorry, ma'am, we didn't consider it necessary, and we didn't think this could happen. The tumor has to come out, but the fever is too high to do the surgery now."

"So, she will go for surgery as soon as her fever goes down? Correct?"

"Yes, she will."

More ice-cold towels and more antibiotics. At least, Sarah was conscious now. She could recognize her mom and the place where she was. It was amazing how much the nurses helped! Ana remembered the nurses who took care of Alex when he had the heart attack and always thought that it takes a special person to be a nurse, not everybody could be so devoted and unselfish.

Ana shook her head, trying to forget that image. When the fever finally went down, not as much as the doctors wanted, but down to a safer level for surgery, Sarah was rushed into the operating room. Ana was told that her daughter would be back in an hour and a half, no longer than two hours. She went back in the room where Sarah's bed was, grabbed her purse, and went to the waiting room. She called Alex and Phillip and talked to them about all the things she had to go through, not complaining, but feeling the need for comfort. It was so good to hear their voices and to forget a little bit about her suffering. Phillip was angry with the way his sister was treated. He asked lots of questions and wanted to come and talk to the doctors. Ana tried to calm him down.

"Mom, why do all these things happen to us, to her? What did we do wrong, that we are so punished?"

"Son, let me talk, please. Ok, thank you. It isn't about 'why' things happen! Some people have more crosses to carry in their lives; some go through life without knowing what life is. It seems like we belong to the first category. It doesn't help to ask 'why,' we just have to deal with it and try to make the best we can with what we have. I know it sounds stupid to you, but this is how I see things."

"I understand, but why us all the time? Mom, I'm sorry to say it, but it is hard for me to accept it."

"I know, son, I love you so much."

"Mom, I feel bad that you have to fight so much and so hard for all of us. I want to be a better son. I promise I will work on it. I have to be the one to bring you more happiness, not only worries. I know how much I hurt you. I promise, again, I will be the son you want to have."

"Everybody goes through something. There is no person on Earth that doesn't, but like I said, for some it is easier than for others. It's more important to concentrate on what we have to do as a family and to help each other. So, you have to help your father with the house and the business while I take care of your sister. Everything will be ok."

"I have to tell you one more time how much I love you."

"Son, I love you more than you think. Take care and see you soon."

Ana called her sister, Sophia, and they talked about everything under the sky, so the time would go faster. And it did; when Ana looked at her watch, she realized that four hours went by. Four hours, when they said—maximum two. Sarah was still in the surgery room.

Ana ran to the nurse's station and asked what was going on, why her daughter wasn't ready. The nurse asked her to be patient and to wait in the waiting area. Ana could see how embarrassed the nurse was, as she had no answer for the mother waiting for her daughter to come out of surgery.

Ana went back to the waiting room, grabbed a notebook that she had in her luggage, and tried to write down things that happened in her life. She always wanted to write about her grandparents, her parents, so her children would know who their ancestors were and the history of their family, but working so many days, so many hours, she never had the time to sit down and write down her memories.

She didn't have more than a few old pictures, at least, not enough to put together a family tree. Ana's mother gave her the pictures left behind by previous generations, most of them with no inscriptions on the back. Ana remembered her mother saying that most of the documents and pictures had been destroyed during the Second World War and asked her to save them. And Ana took care of those pictures, she framed and treasured them.

So, there wasn't much to show her children, but she could feel she had a moral obligation to write about, at least, what she remembered. The words wouldn't have "a meeting" in her mind. The words weren't coming; they refused to be put together. She tried a few times and realized her mind was functioning only for Sarah.

Time was working against Ana's patience; there were so many

waiting hours. Nobody came to talk to her, to let her know the situation of her daughter and to explain why it took so long—why she was still in the operating room after eight hours. She could feel gray hairs growing, her whole body was getting bent towards the ground, and her spine was nonexistent. Ana's body was cold like a stone.

Suddenly, the door opened and a bed was rolled in. Sarah was lying in that bed with tubes coming out of her, all over her body! Ana knew that horrible image would never leave her mind for the rest of her life. "What happened to my daughter? Is she alive? What are those tubes for?"

"Ma'am, please, calm down, she's alive."

"You tell me to calm down? Almost nine hours, nobody came to talk to me and to tell me what was going on. Tell me now, right now, what happened to her? Why does she has all those tubes and that bloody bag?"

"The doctor will be here in a few minutes and she will explain everything. We don't know anything; we only brought the bed here, to the recovery room. Sorry, ma'am." They left Sarah and her mother alone.

Ana didn't know where to look first: an oxygen mask covering Sarah's face, tubes connected to a plastic bag full of red liquid that looked like blood coming out of the blanket covering her. She almost started pulling her hair out. Ana was talking aloud, asking herself questions, "What did they do to her? Why so many hours? Did they find cancer and had to remove the tumor? God, have mercy. If I was weaker, I could have a heart attack seeing my daughter like this. God, take care of my baby; she suffered so much all her life. I am not asking you 'why,' but you have to take care of her. I cannot do more than I did; she is in your hands, God, please, look down and see what I see now."

Two doctors came and started talking to Ana.

"Ana, this is the doctor that fixed Sarah's bladder, Dr. Olson."

"What does 'bladder' mean? She had no bladder problems!"

"I know, but this is what happened. I started removing the tumor on Sarah's uterus and the tumor had very deep, strong roots. I tried really hard, but when I did it, I put a hole in Sarah's bladder. I had to stop the surgery and call a urology surgeon. Dr. Olson did an amazing job, fixing the hole. What you see, all those tubes are necessary for the drainage of the bladder. I firmly believe Sarah will have no bladder issues. The tubes have to stay in for at least three weeks."

"Now I understand. Is she going to be ok? Is she going to be here, in the hospital, all these three weeks, or she can go home?"

"You see, because Sarah cannot walk, she needs to be turned from one side to the other, have her wound stuffed with silver sheets."

"What wound? You said it would be laparoscopic! Why?"

"The doctor had to make a twelve-inch incision in order to fix the bladder, the hole in the bladder. The incision looks like a higher C-section scar. Sarah will wake up soon, and the nurses will take care of her. I am so sorry, Mrs. Ana, I am really sorry. Sarah had enough; she didn't need more suffering, or you either. I did my best. Actually, I wasn't able to remove the roots of the tumor. I hope it will never grow back."

"Ok, I understand; we are all just human beings."

"I will be in the hospital for the next twenty-four hours and I will stop by to check on Sarah, your beautiful daughter. See you soon."

The doctors left and Ana didn't move one inch from Sarah's bed. When she woke up, she looked at her mother and asked question after question.

"Sarah, you will be ok, I promise. The doctors did a very good job, and they will check on you shortly."

"Doctors?"

"Yes, you had two doctors; you should know by now how special you are."

Sarah tried to smile and the way she looked at her mother was a hopeless look, a very painful look. She closed her eyes and tears were coming down her cheeks. The worst part was that Sarah had no idea about the incision, about the hole in her bladder, about all the tubes that had to be there for three weeks.

Ana thought about how she could move her daughter from one side to the other after she took her home. In the hospital, she would have help from the nurses, but in Sarah's apartment?

The next morning, when the doctor visits started, there were lots of med students, doctors, nurses—the room wasn't big enough for all of them.

Ana was tempted to go outside and let the doctors do their teaching, being a university and teaching hospital, but she decided to stay and listen to what they had to say about Sarah's condition.

It was a rare case for the students, and even for some of the doctors. To see a patient that had cerebral palsy, not being able to stand or walk and having all those tubes, the drainage bag, the incision; this wasn't something they would see every day. The visit lasted forever. Everybody had questions to ask and the teachers were glad to show their knowledge. Ana noticed how many times the word "rare" was mentioned during the doctor's visit, and her prayers were quiet and intense.

A few days went by and both Sarah and her mother became more familiar with the horrible view: the tubes and the bag.

Sarah's recovery was slow, way too slow, and made Ana wonder why this happened; why her daughter wasn't getting better faster. She remembered how fast Sarah recovered after her childhood surgeries and she'd had a lot of them. Ana said that one day, she would count how many scars Sarah had from all the surgeries.

The nurse came to take a blood test again, to check what the doctor ordered.

Ana could feel Sarah's body was warmer than normal and she had to cover her with a blanket because she said she was cold.

The results came back—MRSA! For a moment, Ana didn't realize the verdict and she was calm and exhausted, but suddenly she understood the diagnosis. It was a deadly Staph infection. Her body couldn't move, her mouth couldn't say one word, her breath stopped, her eyes were wide open, but they couldn't see a thing. Her mind could only race. *God, this is a deadly condition. God, don't take my daughter away. She did nothing wrong; take me, please!*

What can I do; what can the doctors do?

"Nurse, are you sure this was her blood? Are you sure it is MRSA? Sarah is too weak after the surgery to be able to fight this terrible infection. Tell me it wasn't her blood results. Tell me this is not real—tell me she will live."

"Ma'am, it is her blood test result and we will do everything in our power to save her. Being young, she can fight the infection."

Sarah's condition deteriorated from one day to the next. No medication was strong enough to kill the deadly bacteria. The fever wasn't going down. Ana noticed the doctors getting together, sharing ideas, suggesting different medication, IV antibiotics.

Ana realized how serious the situation was. She noticed how they were talking with low voices and saw them lifting their shoulders like nothing more could be done!

* * * *

"Alex, is Phillip home? I need to talk to both of you."

"I am so glad you called. We miss you here."

"Alex, the situation is very bad. Sarah's infection is so strong that there are no medications to work against this horrible disease. The doctors tried everything they knew, and I can see how disappointed they are."

"You seem like you are giving up on Sarah!"

"What? I will never give up on my daughter. I've been constantly saving her life from the day she was born, but this time, I lost my strength. I need you and Phillip. I need a shoulder to cry on. Why did I leave my country? I had all my relatives there, and they care about us; they love us so much. I have my sister, but she is far away."

"Ana, Phillip and I will be there in two, three days. I have to leave things in order for the business and to make arrangements for the dogs. Phillip can take some time off from what he does now."

"Alex, it is selfish, what I said. No, you have so many responsibilities at home. The girls need you for supplies, equipment and a lot more. I know. You better stay home, and I will let you know how Sarah is doing and if they can find something to save her life. I will take care of her and God will do his job; pray for us."

* * * *

Ana sat close to Sarah, holding her hand.

A priest came into the room and started praying, reading from the Scripture.

Sarah's eyes opened in surprise and she turned her head towards her mother, asking questions without speaking.

Ana was shocked by the priest's appearance and angry that nobody warned her about him coming. She wanted the priest to come and pray for her daughter, but Sarah shouldn't see this. Now, Sarah would feel sure she was dying. The priest should have come when Sarah was sleeping.

After he left, Sarah looked at her mother and said, "Mom am I dying? I don't want to die yet. I'm still young!"

"Sarah, don't talk like this! What you just saw is a standard procedure and it is done in all the hospitals in the country. The priests come and bless the patients, praying for all of them. He wasn't here for you only; he came for all the patients, and I am glad he did. He blessed me too and it feels so good. I saw him blessing the nurses' stations and praying for all the doctors and all the personnel working here. I think it was quite touching."

"Ok. I thought he came especially for me."

"What? Do you think you are that important? No, baby. Let's be grateful for his prayers. Now, get some rest, and I will be here when you wake up. Sarah, your papa and your brother asked me to hug you. My sister said hello. You are young, beautiful, and strong, and you are going to fight this fever. Ok, sleep now. I will rest, too."

A few minutes after Sarah feel asleep, the door opened, and a nurse quietly asked Ana to come outside the room so she wouldn't disturb Sarah.

Ana looked at her daughter to be sure she was sleeping and went outside, walking cautiously.

"Ma'am, I am so sorry to interrupt your quiet time, but I have to talk to you about your daughter's situation."

"Is something wrong? More than it is?"

"The doctors want to talk to you. Would you like to follow me to their office, please?"

Ana followed the nurse and entered the doctor's office.

"Please, have a seat. I need to talk to you about Sarah's condition. We have tried everything possible to get the fever down and get rid of her infection. Nothing has worked, and I have to let you know about it."

"The way you talk, it makes me think that my daughter is dying?"

"I didn't say that. I only say that we have no other options to try."

"Doctor, it is impossible to not find a cure for MRSA! We live in the twenty-first century, and we explore space, the Universe and we don't have the right medication for an infection? It is too much for me to believe. This country is the most powerful in the world; you have to find something to save my daughter. You have to. Help her, please." Ana left the doctor's office holding her daughter's death sentence on her shoulders heavy like a stone.

When she entered Sarah's room, Sarah was still lying down on her bed, and Ana realized she wasn't prepared to answer Sarah's question, she had no time to prepare an answer.

"Where have you been? I thought you went back home."

"How could I leave you? How could you think like this? I went to the bathroom. I am glad you're up though. Let's eat something."

"I am not hungry. I cannot eat."

"I know, but you have to eat in order to get better."

"You did the same thing with Papa, am I right?"

"Yes, and he got better fast and now he is cured. So, open your mouth and eat."

Sarah had to do what her mother told her to do; she was so grateful.

Ana was informed by the nurse that all the doctors would hold an emergency meeting to talk about the most difficult cases and try to come up with suggestions.

Sarah's case was on top of their list. One of the doctors suggested a new trial program that seemed to be promising. That doctor asked permission to start the special IV treatment on Sarah immediately.

All of the doctors agreed because they had attempted all the other options they had. This was their last resort. At least, they would try to save her life one more time.

The doctor came into the room, introduced herself, and started the IV treatment right away. She explained to Ana and Sarah that the treatment was a trial and she was convinced it would improve Sarah's condition.

After she inserted the needle in Sarah's vein, she removed the blanket that covered Sarah's body and washed her long, deep incision with the most powerful antiseptic substance.

Sarah's eyes widened with a silent scream! What a strong girl!

Ana thought she would hit the floor if this were happening to her. After the doctor washed the wound, she cut a silver sheet and inserted it all the way into Sarah's incision.

This was more than Ana could bear! She had to hold the bedframe and find a chair to sit down. It was absolutely barbaric— at least, it looked like that.

Before the doctor left, she hugged Ana and kissed Sarah on her forehead, then said, "Sarah, this new treatment will make you feel better. See you later. I will stay here with you to follow the treatment, step by step. Mrs. Ana, if you need me, I will be outside at the nurse's station."

"Thank you, Doctor. I don't think I could handle what you just did."

"Actually, as soon as Sarah feels better, you will be the one stuffing the wound, but we'll talk later about that. First, we want to see that fever go down."

* * * *

The fever did go down, one point a day, and this was a sign of success. The doctors' expressions were happier and they brought the whole team to see the "miracle!" It was the term they used when teaching the medical students, explaining all the efforts they put in to save Sarah's life.

Sarah's bladder was working normally and the recovery was smooth, without complications. It was the "wound" that took longer to heal, being in a part of the body that wasn't exposed to air. The silver sheets were worth the money Ana spent. It was hard to "push" those sheets inside the incision, but Ana got stronger and she knew she had no other choice.

Ana took care of her daughter, day and night, for an entire month. The incision started to heal, the bladder was working normally, and they had a check-up appointment coming soon.

"Sarah, we're going to have the check-up appointment in a few days. I hope the doctor will give us the green light, so we can go home. Or, maybe it would be better to go to Florida so you can recover there!"

"What about your clients? How can you come with me?"

"God took care of this! All this time I spent with you, and I was away from the business, the girls I work with took care of all the clients, making them happy. I checked with my girls, and it seems that everybody is happy. The clients love my girls as much as they love me."

"I don't believe it, but if you can miss few more days, good for me. I would love to go to Florida. Mom, we went through a lot together."

"Yes, we did!"

The appointment went better than they thought. The doctor gave Sarah permission to go home and recommended another check-up in two months.

Ana was so happy that she wanted to jump up and hug the doctor, but she made efforts to be calm. She took Sarah back to the apartment and called Alex right away. She could hear the screaming over the phone; he was so happy to have them come home again.

Phillip couldn't hold his happiness; he wanted to get in the car and come and take them home. But it was such a long way and Sarah's fresh wounds needed a smooth ride to not hurt her.

Escape

The recovery time was the most wonderful time for the entire family. The sun, the sound of the waves, and the love they had for each other made them feel happy and blessed, and they were.

Alex's cancer was still in remission, Sarah was feeling better, the business was going smoothly, and Phillip was in love.

CHAPTER SEVENTEEN

"Mom, I would like you to meet Kate, my girlfriend. May I bring her home? Actually, she knows you."

"What? Is she my client?"

"No, but she was in our home a long time ago."

"Did you say 'a long time ago'? So, why didn't you introduce her then?"

"It is a long story. Mom, I really like this girl. She's smart and so, so, so beautiful. She is tall and thin. I love her. I hope you will like her because I want you to get along with her. I know you get along with everybody. No, I take it back. I remembered how much you tried to like one of my girlfriends, but it was impossible. It was an exception coming from you."

"That is true. I am kind of an easy-going person, but if something doesn't go with my instinct, there's no chance for me to like that person, and she was one of them. I hope that history will not repeat itself. Tell me more. It seems that this young woman got your heart and this makes me so happy. I can say that things have started to fall into place, finally. You will make a beautiful couple; I know it. You know what I am going to say as soon as you get married!"

"Of course, I know… 'give me lots of grandchildren,' am I right?"

"Like always, you are right. At least you know what you have to do to make me happy. Your father will be the best grandfather in the world. I will be too, but I have to discipline, to teach the right things. And kids don't like that, but they will love me, for sure, because I will have good food to offer."

They laughed together and had a good time, trying not to think about the time when Sarah had to go back to her apartment and continue with her life, her independent life. But that time came, and the entire family took Sarah to the airport where they hugged each other like they knew the end of the world was coming.

Sarah was overwhelmed by her family's love and sacrifice. "I have the best family. We love each other so much. I got used to being with you every day, Mom, and it will be hard to go to the apartment and be alone again. I don't think there are many parents like you. You give everything for your children; you both live for your children. I am so blessed to have you. I love you." She cried and smiled and her tears were saying more than her words. "Phillip, don't forget to invite me to your wedding!"

"Are you crazy? You will be part of her brides' team. I don't know all the names—you know cause it's girlie stuff!"

"Ok, I'll wait for the invitation."

The plane took Sarah to her world. A different world, but a much better world! She had wings; she could go to college, do volunteer work, see Manhattan, movies, libraries, museums. She could enjoy life like anybody else.

Phillip was busy with his life, spending time with the love of his life.

Ana loved Kate! When she met her for the first time, she was speechless. That girl had such a posture; she had something that was telling Ana: *"I know who I am; I know I am beautiful and smart; and I love your son."*

Ana noticed that it would take time to make this girl love her; they were different, and their presentation was different. Ana was a hugger while Kate was reserved and polite, waiting to be conquered. Ana respected Kate's position. Time made them good friends.

"Mom, I'm very happy with Kate. I love her."

"I'm happy too. You made the right decision and I cannot wait to see you both married."

"What do you mean 'both'? Is Sarah getting married too?"

"No, she just rejected her boyfriend."

"What? He loves her so much. What happened?"

"Your sister told me that her boyfriend isn't what she wants. He will move out soon. His mother adores your sister and her heart is broken. I have no right to intervene or to try to convince her. It is her life, not mine."

"Yes, it is her decision. You are right to not get involved. You do get involved a lot, but not in her private life."

"Tomorrow, I'm going to call her again and see what's new with her. Hopefully, her health is better. I don't think I can take anymore. What a life. Son, I should write a book about how many things we went through together, am I right? I know I should, but it is hard to write a book in a language that is not your first one. You never know, maybe the time will come one day."

"Mom, call me after you talk to my sister. I want to know how she's doing."

"I will, son. Love you, and take care; make me happy."

Ana let a few days pass, then grabbed the phone to talk to her daughter—but first, she prayed to God to hear good news. "Hi, Sarah, how are you?"

"Oh, I am so glad you called. I keep going to my classes, but I cannot pass the lab. Hopefully, the teacher will understand that I cannot dissect an animal or insects. My hands don't work like other people's hands. My left hand is almost dead. It is so difficult for me."

"Of course, it is, but keep trying. What about mathematics?"

"Mom, I thought I loved you, but when you ask me about mathematics, I don't love you."

"I got it, and it is normal to be hard for you. You didn't go to school like all the other kids, so we were glad to see that you learned something. We are grateful that you can speak, think and we consider you a normal person, with or without mathematics."

"Thank you, Mom, you made me feel better."

"Are you still volunteering for the American Red Cross?"

"I do, of course! Next month, you're invited to participate in an award ceremony. I will be one of the recipients."

"Oh my God, this is such an honor! We'll be there to celebrate together. I am so proud of you. It will feel good to be in New York for a celebration, not only sad things."

Ana hung up the phone and told Alex how happy she was. She had sparkles in her eyes, making her look beautiful. Alex noticed right away. Ana's face reflected so much of her soul that she could never have a job that required having a frozen face.

"Next month, we go to New York!"

"Is Sarah sick again?"

"No, thank God, she's doing well. Do you remember the American Red Cross, where she has volunteered for years?"

"I remember how much she enjoys going there."

"Well, she will receive an award for her dedication and hard work. Isn't she an amazing young lady?"

"Yes, she is. I am happy for her. I love when we get good news, finally."

Alex and Ana went to New York to be with Sarah for her happy moment. They brought a huge bouquet of flowers and took a taxi directly to the ceremony place. Sarah received three certificates for different accomplishments. The night was a series of laughter, happy tears, and pictures. If only life would be like this all the time.

Once they got back home, Alex and Ana had to go directly to work, because their business was getting busier and busier. It was an unbelievable thing, to see your business grow like this. Hard work and honesty was their motto and it paid off. Literally. Ana's coworker decided to purchase the business and the deal was made.

Alex couldn't contain his glee. "I cannot believe I will live close to the ocean and go fishing! Are you sure this is real?"

"I'm not sure I will be happy there. I have started having hot flashes, and the heat won't help me. But this is my way to show you my love. I do it for you, and I know I will find my way around. Who doesn't love the ocean? I must be crazy to answer differently than millions of people. Ok, let's move there and start a new, and hopefully, a much better life. You deserve it."

"You have no idea what this means for me; thank you."

* * * *

The house they owned for so many years was waiting for them to live there, to be happy. Nobody liked the "moving" part of starting a new life, but it was part of it. They kept the house they had in Atlanta for a while, and moved to the most beautiful part of Florida.

"Alex, do you remember me saying that my best medication is being busy?"

"How could I forget such nonsense?" he teased.

"Ok, so that being said, I would like to start a new business, similar with what we had in Atlanta, but here in the Sunshine State. What do you think about it?"

"What? No, we are too old for this."

"No, we can still do it. So, let's get started."

Alex knew it was a "no win" situation. If she wanted to work, she would work—no questions asked.

In two weeks, they found a place and Alex was able to put together a space where his "crazy" wife could work, doing what she loved the most...providing beauty treatments. He tried to show her the cruel reality of starting a business without knowing anyone. "You don't know one person. How do you think you can make it?"

"Alex, how many people did I know when we started the other business we had? None. Quality work and honesty speak for themselves. But I cannot do anything without you, like always."

Alex knew there was something in his wife's eyes that made people trust her. Her smile was contagious. He knew Ana would soon feel like she had the spa forever. He worked twenty hours a day and hired some help for work that needed licensing and insurance. Alex did a beautiful job, and after getting all the papers in order, the spa was opened.

Ana went to all the businesses around her location to let them know about the new beauty place. Soon she had article in a local magazine, so people found her quickly. Phillip came and helped his father again.

What a joy to see father and son working together. It was the harmony in their relationship, with few words but lots of love.

"Son, how is Kate? I wish to see her here."

"She'll come; don't worry. She's such a great girl, Mom. I love her."

"I'm so glad to see you in love! Doesn't it feel good?"

"How do you know?"

"What? Do you think I don't love your father? Why did I marry him?"

"I know and it shows sometimes, but most of the time, it's just work, work."

"Wait till you get married, and then you tell me how it can be done without work."

* * * *

Phillip and Kate got married. What an amazing wedding; what a celebration!

Love was in the air...love was everywhere.

Ana felt like her life was just beginning with her son's wedding. Now she imagined having grandchildren and taking care of them.

Sarah was the happiest she could be that her baby brother was getting married. Phillip's wedding was the highlight of Sarah's life. After the wedding, Sarah joined her parents in Florida to spend a few more days together. There were so many hours to chat. It was a happy time. Ana was happy to see her family together.

"Mom, I'm friends with an old gentleman. He lives in the same building with me, on a different floor."

"Old, how old?"

"A lot older, but it feels so good to have somebody to talk to, to not be alone all the time. I'm glad to have somebody to go places with, to have dinner."

"Sarah, I'm glad you have a friend, but if you get attached to this person, it will be really hard for you when his time comes."

"I know."

"At least, don't say I didn't warn you. It will be very hard for you." Ana knew her daughter was ok now, but soon, when the gentleman would be gone from this world, Sarah would be devastated. It was her choice and Ana decided to not spoil the short time they had together.

* * * *

Two more years went by and life couldn't be better. The children were ok, healthy; the business was growing and Ana worked hard for wonderful results. The family was getting together to celebrate the holiday every Christmastime. Ana purchased a ticket for Sarah lasting a full month, to spend time together. They went to pick her up from the airport, and Ana couldn't wait to see her beautiful daughter. When she arrived, Ana was delighted to see how good her daughter looked. Sarah was feeling good; you could see it in her eyes.

"We're so happy to have you here. Your brother and Kate will be here shortly so we can spend a wonderful holiday together as a family. Sarah, you look really good."

"Thank you, Mom, but look how wonderful Papa looks! He is so tan!"

"He is tan and, thank God, healthy. This is the most important thing. I am watching his health like an eagle."

"Mom, I'm happy Papa looks so good."

"What about me?"

"You know the answer! I love you. You are so beautiful, and I hope to look like you one day."

"Your brother is so handsome also. Sarah, we have nice-looking men around us; we are lucky."

Phillip and Kate arrived late that afternoon and the house was full of happiness and love. The holiday brought gifts, music, good food and the time flew by. They were talking and sharing events from their daily lives. Ana almost forgot to bring more food to the table, her heart had been so full with what she was seeing. She would treasure the image forever.

A few days after, Phillip and Kate went back to their home, back to work. Phillip called from the road to thank his parents again and tell them how much they, he and Kate, enjoyed the time spent together.

* * * *

Alex and Ana found a small church, far away, but that church was giving them the peace and love they needed. The church was a Christian Orthodox, the people were very friendly, and you could feel how much they cared about everybody. The atmosphere was pure and blessed. Ana said numerous times how touched she was by the Holy Spirit. She never felt like this before.

They took Sarah with them to attend the church service every time she visited. Sarah was surrounded by love and care; everybody was so attentive. She liked the fact that there were lots of infants and toddlers in the church. Sarah always loved children. The priest was kind and had passion for his preaching.

One Sunday, after the New Year, the family was coming back from the church. They stopped to have lunch, they did some shopping, and, on the way back home, Sarah said, "I will call my friend to see how he's feeling. When I left, he didn't feel good; he had pneumonia."

When she called him, nobody answered. She was worried. "I will call the hospital."

Sarah called the admissions desk of the hospital close to their apartment building.

After a few calls, she was told that her friend had passed away. Sarah turned the phone off and couldn't stop crying for hours. Finally, she said, "He's dead. Why did I leave him alone? Why did I come here? I should have stayed with him; he was so sick."

"Sarah, this isn't your fault. He was an old person; he got sick. Do not blame yourself, please."

Sarah was devastated. When she was able to talk, she said that she had to go back to New York for her friend's funeral.

"I understand, and I'll go with you so you won't be alone."

"Thank you, Mom. I appreciate it."

Ana was so tempted to say. *"I told you this would happen, "* but she didn't want to hurt Sarah more than she already was. "Sarah, I will stay with you for the funeral, then I'll go back to the airport right after. Do you remember that I have a few things to finish? I need to get back quickly. I wish I could stay longer, but I know that somebody will give you a ride back from the cemetery to your apartment. I understand you have to be there."

"Mom, I am so sorry that you have to fly in such weather. You have to call me as soon as you get home, promise?"

"I will call, of course. I was thinking that I spend more time in New York than I do at home! But I have only one daughter, and I love her. I call my mission 'love care' as it seems to be my name."

"Mom, I will never let you be in a nursing home! I will take care of you."

Ana wanted to ask Sarah how could she take care of her when she was in a wheelchair and the one who needed help, but she thanked her daughter for being so concerned.

"I love the name 'love care' it is the same way I feel about you and my papa."

Ana looked at her daughter with so much love that she got tears in her eyes, tears of love. *Why did we move from this city and leave Sarah alone? Did we do the right thing? It is my own fault, only my fault. I was the one with the idea of moving. I tried to have a better, safer life for our son and for us; what about Sarah? My whole life I refused to put my child in a special category. I wanted her to be 'normal,' to have a normal life! This was our reason for coming to America. This country gave Sarah the tools to become an independent woman, but like all of us, we are born with a 'road life, a destiny' that only God can stamp our lives with. This destiny is stronger than any country in the world; it is our fate. I shouldn't blame myself for what happened in Sarah's life, but I do! I feel I am responsible for everything. Ok, you didn't come here to have debates with yourself; you are here to help Sarah get through the funeral and give her the emotional support she needs. Get your mind together and start working.* She tried to get rid of all her anxiety.

Alex took them to the airport, thinking how hard it would be for his *girls*, as he liked to call them, to face such a sad event. He knew he would have to be alone again. He was really sad for his wife that she had to fly so often to New York to help their daughter. But it was a fate they didn't choose.

Sarah and Ana arrived at New York on a cloudy, freezing day. Ice was everywhere, and huge amounts of snow were pushed against the sides of the roads making traffic impossible. But for Ana, it was just another trip to the big city, to help her daughter. Sarah opened her apartment door and was speechless: everything was upside down looking like she'd been robbed!

Ana ran to the security desk asking for help. They came and checked the apartment then suggested that Sarah call the police.

Sarah told her mother that she remembered she'd left a key with one of her friend's relatives. The moment that person found out about the death of her relative, she must have gone to Sarah's apartment looking for a will or money—at least, this is what came up in Sarah's mind. So, she decided to not file a police report.

Ana couldn't leave her daughter in such a mess, and she started putting things back where they belonged. It was a really good thing for Ana's mind. She worked so hard that she hadn't even realized how fast the day was gone. At least Sarah's apartment was functional again.

Being in a wheelchair, Sarah couldn't lift the heavy things, so she couldn't be more grateful than she was. "Mom, you saved me again! 'Thank you' will not be enough, Mom. I love you."

"I know, my dear. This is what mothers are made for."

"No, you aren't right about that. I heard my colleagues complaining about their parents, a lot. Some of them don't even talk to their parents."

"Sarah, you always have to listen to both sides!"

After the funeral, Ana kissed her daughter and said goodbye.

Sarah started crying. She would miss her mom.

"Life goes on, Sarah. Remember, you have a future to take care of. Stay healthy. The best thing to do after what happened to you is to keep yourself extremely busy with school, volunteering, cooking, and cleaning, whatever you have to do. A busy mind is a happy mind. At least, this works for your mom and hopefully, it will work for you too. I wish you would go to church like we do, but this is something that will come naturally to you; nobody can force you. Faith is something you have and I know this, but being in God's place, it will give you a special feeling, a different kind of peace that will fulfill your soul. The time will come. It will, for sure. You have the love for God in your heart; it is only covered in worries and pain. Let it shine. Let that love show its power. Ok, I talked too much, and this isn't my normal thing to do. Let me kiss you again. Take care; I love you."

"Goodbye, Mom. Have a safe trip and call me."

Ana left and her heart felt heavy yet again, for leaving her daughter alone. Sarah needed comfort; she loved her friend very much. Ana had a feeling that her daughter would have a tough time after losing the man she was attached to. Spending most of her time alone, Sarah had begun to feel like she had a chance to be happy, having company all day long. She was coming home to somebody. Her apartment had life again. Of course, she knew that, after giving up her boyfriend of five years, she would face loneliness, but she preferred it that way, thinking that it wouldn't be so hard. She was wrong and now, she knew it! Loneliness was poison, depression and it can make severe changes in somebody's mind and heart. The older gentleman had filled that gap; he gave Sarah what she needed.

Ana never understood how a young woman could be with an old man, but now she could see how much it meant for her daughter. It was a soul meeting another lonely soul; they united in loneliness, creating calm and peace.

Sarah would now be depleted of her calm and peace, and this would hurt a lot. Ana talked to God during her entire flight, knowing how much help Sarah would need. She was happy to be home again, but her mind was busy thinking of Sarah.

"I am so glad to have you back!" Alex said. "How is Sarah doing?"

"Not so good, but let's hope time will heal her soul wounds. Alex, I had no idea how much our daughter loved that man. I'm not sure 'love' is the right word, but she was very attached to him. She told me how they were spending time together, how he would wait for her when she was coming back from school or her activities. She was never alone, and this made her feel safe and loved. It made her feel like a woman."

"I understand, though, I never thought about it. It does make sense, but I don't understand why she let her boyfriend go. He was even younger than Sarah and so much in love with her. Well, it seems like it isn't my territory. I better stick with my tools!"

Ana laughed. "You're right; this is a woman thing, and we have more sensitive feelings."

"This I know."

* * * *

Phillip was doing well and his beautiful, gorgeous wife was just an angel sent by God. They had a nice home decorated with taste and love.

Ana could sense love in everything she touched or looked at. Yes, Ana had a special feeling for this word, and maybe this was the reason she wouldn't use it too often. But when she did use the word "love," it made all the sense in the world; it had a different power— a different feeling.

Ana was working hard to keep the business running and to make her clients happy.

She had so many "projects" for Alex that he almost didn't feel like he was retired. Ana knew how to keep him from being bored! They both laughed every time she said it.

The dogs they got for their son were amazing company. Ana and Alex didn't have friends, as it was something they never had time for. To have really good friends, you had to spend time together, doing things together, exchanging visits, and they never had that necessary time. Their friends were their family. Ana knew this wasn't a good thing; people needed people. When she looked back at their life, she saw there was never time for socializing, for friendship. There was always something to do, someone to help, somewhere to go, to take care of somebody in the family, or maybe, and this seemed to be closer to the truth, they had no desire to let somebody else enter their circle.

Everything they did, all their lives, had been done together. Now, it was way too late to become friends with people they knew in passing. Again, the family loved being like this.

Ana and Alex had their hands full and this made them grateful and happy. Both of them knew they would have plenty of time available for a grandson or a granddaughter.

The dogs knew whenever something wasn't right. They especially, knew when one of them was unhappy or sick. They were excellent family members and Alex and Ana loved them a lot.

When Sarah came to visit, the dogs would stay under her wheelchair the whole time. Their dogs had skin problems and Ana would give them pedicures, skin massages, and make special lotions to rub on their skin. When they saw Ana coming through the door, they became crazy! Being English bulldogs, jumping or moving that much made Ana afraid that the dogs would have heart attacks! It made her happy to see how much love the dogs had for her.

She needed love; it was too much for her to see her daughter devastated. Ana loved everything about her home, even if she'd wanted to sell it a long time ago. It made her feel like she was in paradise; the home had a soul! Although, she always wondered why the locals didn't go to the beach? Remembering when she and Alex were coming for weekends only, the first thing they did, the very next morning, was go to the beach and walk along the shore. It was the best treatment for relaxation; the best thing they could do for themselves in order to go back to work full of energy. Once they moved to the ocean, though, they stopped going to the beach. Ana would take Sarah when she visited, to enjoy the ocean's sounds and the salty air. It was the best thing to do, being together in paradise.

* * * *

Soon after the New Year celebration, the phone rang. It was Sarah, and she was frantic. "Mom, I'm afraid somebody will kill me. Mom, I hear voices saying that Phillip will be killed. Mom, call our relatives from Romania and see if they are ok because somebody will be killed." Sarah kept screaming, clearly scared to death.

Ana's heart was beating a hundred miles per hour and her body was shaking. "Sarah, please, stop and talk to me, please. What is going on with you?"

"I cannot stay in my apartment! I am going to the emergency

room; I feel safer there."

"You cannot go there; they will put you in the psychiatric section! Please, don't go. Talk to me, please. What is going on? Who is going to kill you? What voices do you hear?"

"I'm leaving. I can't stay here. I am leaving."

"Sarah, promise me you will stay home. Your mom is coming to get you. Promise me, you are not going to leave your apartment. It is ice everywhere and it's dangerous to go with the wheelchair; please, don't go anywhere."

Ana knew right away something horrible happened to her daughter's mind. Something must be bothering her soul badly; she suffered so much after her friend's death. Ana was wondering why she hadn't seen any changes in the year since Sarah lost her friend. How was it possible to be so blind? Ana talked to her daughter almost every day and she could sense a change, but she didn't remember noticing anything specific. It couldn't happen overnight; there were supposed to be some signs. How did she miss them?

"Alex, I have to go to New York now. I know it is extremely urgent. Sarah has lost her mind. She hears voices; she cannot be by herself in her apartment. It is bad, really bad."

Alex didn't say one word. He was speechless. "How many times have we had to save our daughter? What is wrong now?"

Ana packed a few things, and Alex took her to the airport. She was lucky to find a ticket for the last flight of the day. Living so far away from a big city, the flight had to make two stops to get to New York. Ana wished she had wings; she would fly faster than the plane.

The weather was the worst they had seen for many years. Icy roads, snow, rain, all at the same time. The taxi she took wasn't moving because the traffic was very bad. Finally, she arrived at Sarah's apartment; she knocked on the door, no answer.

A neighbor opened her door and recognized Ana. Of course, all the tenants knew her. The lady told Ana that Sarah went to the emergency room, the one closest to their building. "Mrs. Ana, your daughter looked really bad, really bad; she had scared eyes. I never saw her like this. I hope she got there ok. I am so sorry for her; she is such a sweet young lady."

Ana didn't have time for conversations, so she thanked the neighbor and ran towards the elevator. She then had to fight the ice, trying to walk faster, pulling the carry-on behind her. No old person should have to go through this; it was so dangerous. Finally, she arrived at the emergency room and she asked about her daughter, where she was.

Before she received an answer, she saw Sarah sitting in a corner of the waiting room looking frightened. She was moving her eyes from one corner to another, from the floor to the ceiling, and back again, all over the room. She didn't even seem to recognize her own mother.

"Sarah, it is me, your mother! Look at me, please." Ana hugged her daughter and started crying.

"Are you related to Sarah?" a nurse asked Ana.

"Yes, I am her mother."

"I see the resemblance, but I have to do my job. This is the second time she has come to us and was seen by a psychiatrist. The doctor gave her a prescription for antidepressants and she has to get them from the pharmacy. Meanwhile, we gave her some, but it seems like they aren't working. The way she looks is the same. Ma'am, she can't be left alone. The doctor recommended that Sarah be admitted to the psychiatric ward of our hospital. Let me know what you decide."

"Thank you for taking care of her. Let me see if I can talk to her, thank you."

"Oh, I forgot to tell you that she told us that she went to the closest hotel to her apartment building and paid for a room. The charge was half of her monthly income. She got the key, went inside the room, looked around, and left after few minutes, because she was scared somebody was going to kill her. She also said that all her family members will be killed. Ma'am, I am so sorry. I wish I could do more for her and for you."

"Thank you and I appreciate that you took care of my daughter. I can see you are a mother, too. The way you took care of my daughter was more than a nurse's job."

"Yes, I am. And looking at your luggage, I think you're an amazing mother. Something sad must have happened with your daughter that she had such a reaction. Did she have a recent loss?"

"No, it happened almost a year ago, not recently. Do you think it caused such a horrible reaction, after so many months?"

"The mind is a mystery, and it does things on its own. I am so sorry. I so hope it will get better."

"Thank you, again. I will try to make her go home now."

Ana put her scarf around Sarah's neck, to keep her warm, even if the scarf was wet and cold, but it was a touch, so Sarah might look at her mother and talk to her. They went to the apartment and Ana prepared something for them to snack on so Sarah could take her medication.

"Mom, take me home, please, take me home. I will not stay here."

"I will, I promise. Let's go to bed and get some sleep." Ana took Sarah to the bathroom and did as much as she could to get Sarah ready for the night.

When they came back in the room, Sarah asked her mother to sleep on a chair, to not sleep in the bed. Ana was perplexed!

"Please, pull a chair in front of my chair and don't face the window. I will put my chair against the door, so nobody can come and kill you."

"Ok, Sarah, I will do like you said." She pulled up a chair, grabbed a blanket for each of them, turned off the lights, and tried to get some rest.

"Mom, you have to move your chair; you're facing the window."

"Sarah, your windows face an interior court; nobody has access there."

"Mom, please, move your chair."

Ana moved her chair the way Sarah wanted. She put her head in Sarah's lap and she could feel Sarah's nails digging into her arms. "Sarah, I am here with you. I'm not leaving you. I promise I will take you with me. Please close your eyes and try to get some sleep. Good night, I love you."

Sarah and Ana weren't able to close their eyes, each waiting for the day to bring light. Neither of them spoke, but they were both anxious and full of distress.

Sarah's mind was fighting enemies that were trying to kill her and her family.

Ana's mind kept trying to figure out if she should leave New York with Sarah to see a doctor first, or to take Sarah to a doctor first thing in the morning.

Ana's dilemma was solved by Sarah.

"Mom, you promised me that you would take me home to Papa; you promised me. Did you change your mind? They will kill me and all of us."

"I will keep my promise. What if we go and fill the prescription at the pharmacy, so we will have some pills to take, then get a taxi then go directly to the airport? But you have to take the manual wheelchair, so we can fold it for the taxi. It will be really hard to push your wheelchair and my carry-on. The streets are covered in ice, but New York has the best people in the world, they help each other. Somebody will help us, when they see how we struggle."

Ana realized she was trying to make Sarah change her mind and stay in New York for help, for medical care. It was a huge city with multiple solutions, experts, hospitals. Taking Sarah to Florida could be a very stupid thing. They were living in a small city where everything was limited. She would never be able to offer Sarah the kind of care she needed. It was a very serious situation, and she couldn't even talk to her husband and her son. Sarah was next to her all the time, scared to be alone.

My God, how much I need Alex and Phillip. I need them so much; God, help me, tell me what to do.

It seemed that God answered Ana's prayer because Sarah was making the decision for both of them. "Mom, let's go. I cannot stay here. They're coming to kill us."

"Ok, Sarah, let's go."

They left the apartment, went to the pharmacy, got the medication, and Ana gave Sarah the prescribed dose to help her calm down.

People stopped and helped Ana push the wheelchair so they could get to the corner of the street and catch a taxi.

After a while, they finally arrived at the airport. Ana was so relieved to walk on dry ground, no more ice. She approached the ticket counter and asked the clerk to find her a ticket for Sarah and to update the ticket she had already for Florida, Pensacola or Panama City.

"Please, ma'am, we have to leave today. My daughter suffers from severe depression and she is in really bad shape. We have to leave New York today, please." Ana pulled out her return ticket and showed it to the lady she talked to.

"Your ticket is for tomorrow, not for today."

"I know it, but I need to leave today."

The way this mother and daughter looked must have made the clerk's heart melt. Like she couldn't believe how much they suffered; it was so visible. She acted as if she truly wanted to help them. "Let me see what I can do for you. I'll talk to my manager. Stay here; don't go anywhere. I will be back."

"Thank you so much, God bless you."

* * * *

Thirty minutes later, the lady came back and she had a smile on her face. "Ok, this is what I can do for you. You are going to fly to Houston, Texas, and from there, the next morning, take a flight to your destination."

Ana was so grateful to leave the place that was making her daughter so scared. But she also knew that it wasn't the city that made Sarah ill; she knew it was a much deeper issue!

Sarah was calm but she was watching everything around her. When she found out they were going to leave, she had a smile in her eyes. Her mother was keeping her promise.

They arrived at Houston in the middle of the night. It was a huge airport. Ana was pushing the wheelchair and her carry-on trying to find a place where they could eat something. They found a place selling old, cold pizza. Ana sat down and, afraid to leave Sarah alone, asked the man selling pizza to come to their table.

He didn't seem sure why he was asked to go to their table, but he did. Once the man took a look at the women, he looked as if he understood the situation and brought them two slices of pizza.

That cold and old pizza never tasted so good. Even Sarah ate a little. When they finished eating, they went to the gate; Ana found a chair and tried to get some sleep. It was very, very cold, or maybe they felt like this because of being tired. Somebody brought a few blankets. Those blankets were like the best comforters they ever had.

Sarah kept looking around, desperately. She seemed to be scared of everything that moved. It was a night that would never be erased from Ana's memory. Sarah's arms were locked around Ana's hands. The morning came and both were happy to go to the Sunshine State where Alex was waiting for them. Ana called Alex and let him know the time they would get to Pensacola. No details, nothing, because Sarah was next to her the entire time.

"Thank God, you are here," Alex said, putting his arms around his girls. "I was so worried about you flying so far in order to get here, especially with this weather. Sarah, I am so glad to see you; everything will be ok. We need each other; we need our family. It is everything we have, and God is watching over us. You will be ok. I know it. Phillip will take some time off and come here to spend some time with you."

"Is he alive?" Sarah asked her dad without smiling. Any other time somebody mentioned Phillip's name, Sarah would smile and her face would fill with love. Not this time. It was like she hadn't even heard his name.

Alex looked over at Ana, like he couldn't believe what he just heard.

Ana didn't say one word but she put her head down.

Alex then seemed to realize how devastating his daughter's situation was. He kept touching his daughter's head, and Ana could see tears in his eyes.

* * * *

The next morning, Ana took Sarah to a psychiatrist.

The appointment lasted a long time, but it made Ana feel that she could help Sarah right away.

The diagnosis was clear and hard to admit. A severe chemical imbalance in the brain had been caused by extreme stress, and the pain of losing a loved one. But the doctor also admitted that no one could know the real cause for sure. "We have to start treatment right away. This is a serious condition that can have really bad consequences if left untreated. Your daughter has to get counseling, therapy, and medication. Let's hope we can find a medication that works from the beginning."

The doctor was very calm and he didn't seem to be in a hurry, so he asked Sarah about New York, school, volunteer work, and about her friend that passed away. Sarah's answers were clear, and she really enjoyed the conversation with her doctor.

Ana couldn't believe how much different her behavior was! *Is she the same person? She seemed normal, focused and not as scared as she was in New York.* Ana wasn't sure if she should be happy or concerned, so she talked to God in her mind asking him to take care of her baby girl.

The appointment with the doctor was a good thing for both of them. Sarah was less scared and Ana felt like she had somebody she could talk to about helping her daughter. She needed to talk to her husband as soon as they got home.

"Alex, we are now at square one again, the same as the first time we arrived in America."

"What do you mean?"

"Our purpose, our goal was to see Sarah living on her own, so we can leave this world in peace, am I right?"

"Yes, you are right."

"We have a mission, again."

"I know it; we always have a mission…children first."

Ana took Sarah to all the therapy sessions and watched like an eagle over her, to be sure she was safe. The doctor explained to Ana that it is possible for patients with that type of psychiatric condition to commit suicide, or harm somebody. When the weather permitted, Ana took Sarah to the beach, to enjoy the sun. She noticed a huge change in Sarah's look after being in the sun. Ana tried to spend more time with her daughter, and not leave her alone.

* * * *

A young, beautiful lady came one day to the spa where Ana worked. Soon after they met each other, that young lady became Ana's God-sent gift. God knew what Ana needed to be able to be with her daughter and to be the best instrument for Sarah's cure.

Soon, the young lady became Ana's right-hand girl at the spa. She was running the business like it was her own. She was very talented and caught on to all the skills quickly. Ana was more than grateful to have the young lady working with her and she was recommending the new aesthetician to all her clients. By having the extra help, Ana started working fewer days and the rest of the week she was busy with appointments for her daughter.

Things only got better; Sarah tried five different medications until she found one that did the job.

The doctor seemed to have no more doubts. "Oh, you are so lucky, Sarah! Most of my patients try twenty, thirty different medications before they agree with one. You tried only five, and we are on the right way to recovery. I'm pleased with the improvements I've noticed."

"Me too," Sarah said, smiling. "I don't hear those voices anymore."

"What? Are you sure?" the doctor asked Sarah.

"Yes. I'm still depressed, but no more voices."

"You have no idea how much this means for me. As a doctor, I feel the pain of every patient. I'm part of your treatment plan, and I am you. Sarah, you have made my day. Remember to take your medication, even if you feel better. Keep going to the therapy sessions, try to find a support group and I will see you in two months."

Alex was waiting outside, ready to take his girls home, and when they came to the car, he saw huge smiles on their faces. "Why are you so happy?"

"The doctor is very pleased with the improvements he saw in Sarah's condition. Next visit is in two months! Wow! I am so happy. How about we go to Perdido Key or Gulf Shores?"

"When do you want to go?" Alex asked.

"Now, let's celebrate. Being in the sun is the best thing for Sarah and, to be honest, for me too, and I think it will be good for you too."

"Yes, but we have the most beautiful water and sand here; why drive all the way to Gulf Shores?"

"Papa, I wish I could drive. I love being in the car."

"Ok, I got the message. Let's go."

They went to Perdido Key and had lunch in Foley, a beautiful, small town close to Gulf Shores. Ana took Sarah for some shopping at the outlet mall in Foley and they had a really good time there. It was clear to Ana that she made the right decision; her daughter's smile stayed on her face during the trip, making her parents happy. Alex hadn't seen his girls that happy for a long, long time.

* * * *

Summer arrived and it was so much easier to let Sarah spend a few hours in the sun, at the public beach where there was a ramp. The sound of the waves, their rhythmic motion, and the emerald color of the water were working together to be God's medicine for Sarah.

Everybody could see how much better she looked and felt. She was smiling more often, making jokes like before—it seemed like the old, good times were back.

"Alex, I will start looking for places where people with disabilities can live on their own. I wish she could stay with us, but there's no public transportation in our area. Now we take her everywhere she needs to go, but what about later, when we will no longer be here on Earth? You know exactly what I mean. This has been our eternal conversation."

"I know it and I keep looking. I don't see people in wheelchairs where we live. I know there are, but where do they live? I have no idea."

"It seems like I will be on my mission again. When I brought her here from New York, my mission was to get her mental condition better. Now I've gotten promoted to find a good place for her to live by herself. I don't think it will be an easy job, but I have gotten better at searching on the computer now. Do you remember how hard it was when we tried to find the best schools and neighborhoods for Phillip? We drove around town like maniacs. Knowledge is power—I have no idea who said this, but it is so true. I always wanted to learn computers but, back in Romania, when I asked to be accepted for training, the answer was: 'we don't train traitors!' They considered us traitors; what a shame. I loved the country where I was born. I will always love my country, but my adoptive country helped me, and all of us, so much that I am full of gratitude and love for what I now call 'my' country! Now that Sarah is doing so much better, we should find a clean, friendly place where she can be safe and meet people. She needs to live the same way she did for seventeen years in New York. She is living proof that she can do it. I will find a place I am sure."

It took many hours of searching neighborhoods and buildings, but Ana was determined to find the best place for her daughter. Ana's age was making her even more eager to speed up the process of finding a place for Sarah.

Twenty-five miles away from Sarah's parents, there was a very clean, well maintained building with a beautiful landscape and wonderful apartments. Ana couldn't be happier. "Sarah, let's go and take a look at a place for you. Hopefully, you will like it. I checked almost all the buildings with wheelchair accessibility, and this one is, by far, the best. If you like it, you just have to wait till your name comes up on the waiting list."

"Ok, let's go. I love being with you. You know how much I love our home, but I see how hard it is without public transportation. How I wish I could drive. You already bought a van with a ramp for me, but I'm not allowed to drive. Do you remember when I had the test and the doctor told me that I am not allowed to drive because of my spasticity?"

"How could I forget that test? You had so much hope that you could get the doctor's ok to drive. But do you know something, better safe than sorry. Don't think about this anymore. There are buses to take you places."

Ana had already made the appointment to see the apartment, so they got in the car and went to the building.

Sarah made a good impression with the person showing the apartment. You could see how pleased she was to see such a clean, beautiful young lady. The tenants were all seniors, and they made an exception for Sarah to live there because of her handicap. There were a few apartments, adapted for wheelchair users, on the first floor.

As soon as they entered the lobby, Sarah's eyes lit up; she loved it. High ceilings, an elevator, laundry facility, twenty-four-hour security desk, library, activities room, recreation room—it had everything Ana was looking for. "It is a lot bigger than what I had in New York. I love it, but I don't know anybody."

"You'll meet all the tenants and you will make lots of friends. Did you know somebody when you moved to New York?"

"You're right. I wish I had been able to live by myself like before, but I got used to being with you."

"This should be your last worry; you know I will suffocate you with my presence." Ana smiled and hugged her daughter.

"I know you will be there for me when I need it, this I know for sure. I love you, Mom. Papa and you are just amazing parents. How many can do what you do?"

"Yes, but I think we can do so much because we have been blessed with good health—even your papa is in good health now. We are old, but like my doctor said, we are really 'young' old! I thank God every morning when I wake up for this. I say, thank you for waking me up; thank you for everything and take care of my family and friends! I am kind of demanding, but he likes me praying like this; it comes from my heart, not from the books. I will do anything in my power to see you independent, healthy, and happy Sarah. I know you can be independent, and we have to work together in becoming healthy and happy."

A few months went by and Sarah's name came up on the list for the building she liked. What an event! Ana and Sarah arranged the apartment; Kate and Phillip sent beautiful, useful gifts for Sarah to use in her kitchen. She moved into her new apartment—mission accomplished!

Ana felt happy and sad at the same time. Her daughter was part of her happiness. She'd become so used to taking care of her, eating together, going shopping together, and doing everything together. The house would feel "dead" without Sarah. Ana knew she would cry a lot.

Sarah was doing so much better with her depression, no more voices, no more "killings, tortures, violence." The medications worked and Ana was sure Sarah would take them every day.

"Alex, I am going to spend the night with Sarah, to see how she is doing."

"Are you sure? You wanted her to be independent, and now you are going to spend the night with her? Ok, you know better what to do. Maybe you are right to be sure she is doing things the way she is supposed to."

Sarah started to get accustomed to the new environment. She met new people and everybody was very nice to her. She felt safe in that building and she had fewer depression episodes.

"Mom, I think I can live by myself. I love living here, but I still want to spend time with you and Papa."

"Of course, you will. Where we go, you go, when you want. But you have to look for public transportation, to learn how to get places, and the most important thing is to find a place to work or volunteer. Maybe even to finish school. Being active will make you happier, remember again: busy mind, happy mind."

"This is so true and you're right. God helped me so much. I could be dead or in the madhouse. You and Papa have given your lives for me. You have made so many sacrifices for me and for Phillip; your children always came first. Did you ever do something for you? I mean, you and Papa? Did you ever have fun with Papa? Did you ever go places, just the two of you? I don't think so! Mom, Phillip is ok; he has a family now. He loves his wife so much and soon, they will have a baby or more. I'm ok. I'm so much better than when you brought me down here. What if you and Papa go somewhere to relax and see what life is all about?"

"What is wrong with you? I'm all right, and I did nothing for you. It was a mother's job, done with love and care. I will let you go to bed now; talk to you tomorrow. Take your medications and do not forget to pray. God is all that we have; he did everything. And we, your father and I, were only his instruments. Good night, love you."

"Mom, I wanted to tell you this for a long time: I am so sorry that I cannot walk. We could have done so much together."

"In my mind, you walk. You are my precious love. I feel like my mission is completed now, and you are a fighter, too. Look at how many 'events' you survived. The daughter, like the mother. Good night."

Ana had to leave the apartment so her daughter wouldn't see her crying. What an accomplishment! Finally, Sarah was living independently; she got a new lease on life, like her father a few years ago when he entered remission from the deadly cancer he fought.

She got in the car, took a deep breath, closed her eyes, and leaned her head against the car seat. Ana could feel a huge mountain coming down from her body and her mind. She grabbed her phone and called Alex. "Alex, I want to ask you a question."

"Go ahead and ask me as many questions as you want. I hope you are coming home."

"I am coming home; I just got in the car. Sarah is doing great, and this gives me peace of mind; she is back. Do you remember the gospel about 'lost and found,' the son that left his family, trying to live better than at home, and he lost everything he got from his father? It isn't that Sarah left the home because she wanted to, she had to in order to survive, but this is how I feel right now. I found my daughter; she is back, and I am so happy. This is my question for you… Alex, how many vacations did we have in almost half of century of marriage? Can you count, please?"

"Yes, I can, because it would be enough to count on my fingers on one hand, maybe."

"What if we started counting our vacations with the other hand? But wait, maybe we should wait a few more months, to be sure."

"We have always waited a few more months and a few more."

"I know it, but we didn't choose our fate; it was given to us, like I said before. That time will come, one day."

Epilogue

LOVE…CARE

"Alex, I was really far away. Thank you for holding me tight. I am back now. For all the time you held me close to you, my whole life was playing in my mind like a movie. Do you remember how much I wanted to go to college? Now I am sure I can say that I have graduated the "College of Life" cum laude!"

"Yes, I know it." Alex held her tight.

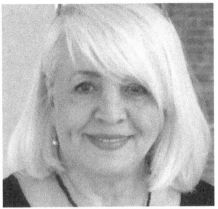

ABOUT THE AUTHOR

G.V. Cora was born in Bucharest, Romania and immigrated to the USA in 1991 with her husband and their two children, one of them being wheelchair bound. Gabriela and her family waited six dramatic years to touch the "promised land."

She became a very successful aesthetician, working hard and as a result, she and her husband, Eugene Voiculescu opened four skincare salons. Three of them in Atlanta, Georgia and one in Miramar Beach, Florida, where they live now. They helped women to achieve high quality skills, to be appreciated and rewarded. Gabriela paid her tribute to the country that adopted her, by becoming a success story.

Her and her husband, Eugene are now happy grandparents of an awesome boy, Liam and they are waiting for one more handsome grandson.

ESCAPE is the follow-up to her 2013 professional publication Skin and Beauty Wisdom, a book full of "tips and tricks" of homemade health and beauty remedies.
G.V. Cora's life is a transition from beauty wisdom to life wisdom.